(7-21-18, 50th!)

Happy Birthday Christine

Medical
AROMATHERAPY

Healing with Essential Oils

KURT SCHNAUBELT

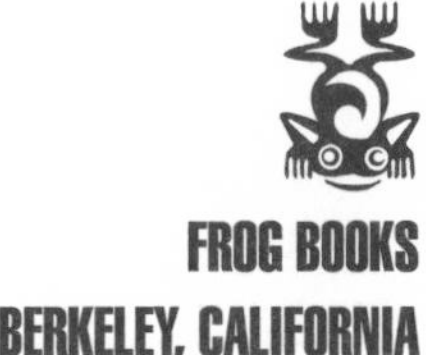

FROG BOOKS
BERKELEY, CALIFORNIA

Published by Frog Books, an imprint of
North Atlantic Books
Berkeley, California

Cover and book design by Andrea DuFlon
Printed in the United States of America

Medical Aromatherapy: Healing with Essential Oils is sponsored and published by the Society for the Study of Native Arts and Sciences (dba North Atlantic Books), an educational nonprofit based in Berkeley, California, that collaborates with partners to develop cross-cultural perspectives, nurture holistic views of art, science, the humanities, and healing, and seed personal and global transformation by publishing work on the relationship of body, spirit, and nature.

ISBN-13: 978-1-883319-69-4

Library of Congress Cataloging-in-Publication Data

Schnaubelt, Kurt
Medical aromatherapy : healing with essential oils / Kurt Schnaubelt
p. cm.
Includes bibliographical references and index.
ISBN 1-883319-69-2 (pbk)
1. Aromatherapy. 2. Medicinal plants. 3. Alternative medicine
I. Title.
RM666.A68S366 1998
615'.321—cd21 97-46512
CIP

11 12 13 14 15 UNITED 21 20 19 18 17

Printed on recycled paper

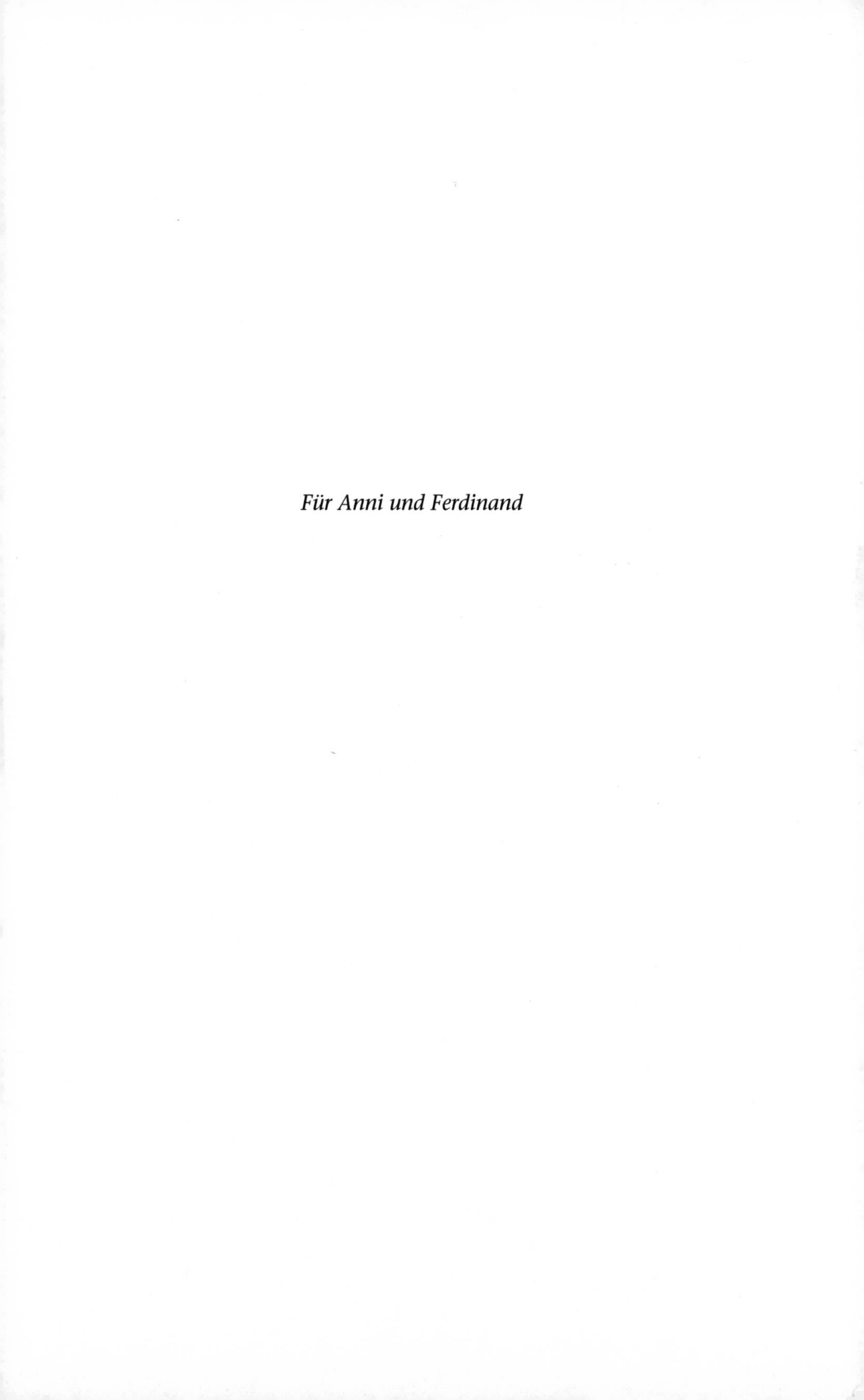

Für Anni und Ferdinand

A Note to the Reader

The material in this book is intended to provide a review of the chemical healing properties of the essential oils of aromatherapy and the socio-cultural context in which medical aromatherapy is situated in 1998. Every effort has been made to provide accurate and reliable information. However, you should be aware that professionals in the field may have differing opinions and change is always taking place. If any of the treatments described herein are used, they should be undertaken only under the guidance of a licensed health care practioner. You and your physicians or licensed health care professional must take full responsibility for the use of the information in this book. The author, editors, and publisher cannot be held responsible for any error, omission, professional disagreement, outdated material or adverse outcomes that derive from use of any of these treatments in a program of self-care or under the care of a licensed practioner.

Contents

Introduction

Aromatherapy is shamanism for everyone. A vote for aromatherapy is a vote to test reality in new ways rather than in a laboratory. With aromatherapy, individual human life plays a role; the life story of a woman or a man receives recognition and respect. The fact that aromatherapy is also a healing tool and a form of communicating with plants is simultaneously part and consequence of the above concept. Subordinating aromatherapy to what can be proven scientifically is either folly or execution of a hostile agenda. The role of science in aromatherapy is clear: it can help us understand some of the more complex mechanisms in which oils can be used to treat symptoms of diseases, but science is *not* equipped to explain the miracles of life to which the interaction with essential oils and plants opens a glimpse.

The total trust that is bestowed on the scientific process is the primary cause for many health problems industrialized societies encounter. Scientific process is allowed to run unchecked and the results are invariably accepted as a blessing even if a sober assessment would have to conclude that some of them are catastrophic. In the health-care sector of society, this process is completely out of control. HMOs routinely subordinate the legitimate health concerns of their customers to profit considerations while legal drugs are causing pathologies and deaths in unprecedented proportions.

All this continues because of the all-encompassing conditioning almost everyone is subjected to from cradle to grave. As children we are told to do what the doctor says, and in high school we are indoctrinated with scientific dogma. Huge institutions are based on producing and administering science, and in public discourse calling something "unscientific" finishes the topic, no further questions asked. Reason has long given way to suicidal commerce. To the same degree, as reason has left the conventional "health"-care drug business, it has become inhuman.

Healing with essential oils is different from purchasing mainstream medical services and products. It is a path away from the hubris of apparatus-medicine. It reverses the current attitudes of commerce before life and information over reason. Aromatherapy is neither destructive business nor brain-dead information management; it embraces all aspects of human life, including instinct and the human spirit. How our shift toward the exclusive dominance of science has dehumanized life in industrialized societies is summed up in a short quotation from Leandis, a Native North American: "Bird has instinct. Humans have reason and instinct. We combine it and make it an emotion. Instinct serves the animal well, but to us it can get in the way, especially if we only react to emotions. The only thing that can interfere with intuition is reason. Reason was humanity's greatest blessing. But not anymore, since it has taken over intuition."

In aromatherapy the chemistry of plants is accepted as a teacher, refreshing our awareness for the wonders of creation. It reverses the sexism of the old system, it approaches health care with intermediate technologies, and to a large degree it liberates us from stifling dependence on cold experts. It returns the power to heal to the layperson. Aromatherapy is a road leading to the mastery of our own health care.

"What we observe is not nature itself, but nature exposed to our method of questioning."
—Werner Heisenberg

ONE

An Unclear Picture

This book sets out to free aromatherapy from the limitations of certain current cultural norms. Aromatherapy does not need to be limited by self-serving, business-minded thinking and the widening gap between scientific reason and a vitalist worldview. Big business threatens to oppress aromatherapy. A new class of "experts"—aromatherapists imitating the conventional system—insists that people are not qualified to take care of their own health. Aromatherapy might grow more rapidly than other alternative methods of healing because it is the most accessible. Aromatherapy easily combines physiological and psychological betterment and, because plants are egalitarian, it does so for poor and rich alike.

Aromatherapy has its basis in the plant organism and its constituent molecules, which possess a chemical intelligence that speaks directly to the human organism. Aromatherapy provides an entirely different outlook on treating disease than the conventional system. Whereas current medicine is highly alienating, fear-based, and believes in the separation of body and soul, aromatherapy seeks to *unite* body and soul, healing our whole being.

What is aromatherapy?

At the end of the twentieth century, the practice of aromatherapy appears to consist of whatever the particular practitioner or user of essential oils might make it to be. Disjointed and scattered, it is a practice without a theory. What definitions exist are massively colored by commercial interests and/or the worldview of those who originate these interests. For instance, conventional scientists who deal with aromatherapy tend to adopt apologetic behavior toward their peers for entering an area as subjective as aroma and human emotions. They correctly realize that many of the observable effects in aromatherapy are very difficult to quantify and therefore are not the stuff from which hard scientific studies are made. The scientist's discomfort around the subject of aroma and emotion is reflected in the attempts to put it in its place by restrictive definitions such as "...such uses of aromatic substances should therefore be called perfume therapy."[1] Mainstream medical disdain for aromatherapy has led many people to believe that its concepts are all nonsense, that only the true scientific-reductionist path can lead to acceptable results.[2] These attempts at defining aromatherapy are obviously driven by the scientific worldview. Commercial interest can be identified when one realizes that science routinely serves corporate interest.

Organizations that educate aromatherapists, especially those that offer certificates or licenses, invest particular authority onto the "experts" of this new profession. Definitions are also offered by grassroots industries in order to "further the cause" of aromatherapy. Their versions often reflect the commercial interests of cottage industries that concentrate on soaps, candles, or other gift-item lines. In the charters of these organizations, the manufacture of such items is considered a valid implementation of aromatherapy. In fact, the by-laws of a North American aromatherapy organization representing mainly such interests delivers a rather precise and well-inspired thesis on what aromatherapy should be to have therapeutic value.

So whose definition is valid? What really *is* aromatherapy? To find reasonable answers to these questions, we will first take a look at the literature.

Aromatherapy's beginnings

Réné-Maurice Gattefossé's *Aromatherapie: Les Huiles essentielles, hormones végétales* was the seminal work published in 1937.[3] It introduced the word "aromatherapy" and created the discipline of therapeutic applications of essential oils. This is not to be confused with the use of aromatic plants, which indeed is as old as humanity. Aromatherapy, however, is a concept inextricably tied to the scientific advances of the twentieth century and the attempts to overcome the fallout of those advances. Aromatherapy is rooted in the Western, industrialized, and science-biased societies of our times. This is reflected in Gattefossé's theories, which put aromatherapy squarely on the basis of modern scientific thought and experimentation. Aromatherapy originated as a medical therapy based on the pharmacological effects of essential oils, which were considered equally effective as the conventional pharmaceutical drugs.

In the first three decades of the twentieth century, chemists learned to identify an increasing number of the components of essential oils. Adhering to the reductionist methodology, clearly the dominant philosophical model to explain the phenomena of nature at the time, researchers searched for "active components" responsible for the oils' physiological actions. Influenced by an exhilarating stream of discoveries that unraveled the chemical composition of essential oils, Gattefossé's aromatherapy was biased toward the concept of active ingredients. Not surprisingly, aromatherapy according to Gattefossé was used to treat a symptom or a disease the same way conventional medicine did. In Gattefossé's approach there really was no division between medicine and aromatherapy; in fact he considered aromatherapy to be an integral part of medicine. But despite the orientation toward pharmacological properties brought about by active ingredients, Gattefossé was also aware of the psychological and neurological effects of essential oils. Integrating these effects into his work, he foreshadowed the holistic approach to aromatherapy that has become dominant today.

The next step in the development of modern aromatherapy came with Jean Valnet's *The Practice of Aromatherapy*, first published in France in 1964.[4] This book catalyzed the popular use of essential oils on a larger scale. Simultaneously addressed to a lay- and medical audience, Valnet presented aromatherapy in a manner very similar to Gattefossé. Twelve years after the publication of Valnet's book in French, it was translated into English and German. Robert Tisserand's *The Art of Aromatherapy* was published in England at the same time, and was the first book to combine a medical approach to aromatherapy with a more esoteric view of essential oils.[5] In 1976, the medical roots of aromatherapy were still weighing in strongly, as even Tisserand described the internal use of medicinal essential oil blends, a notion that has since been reversed by this influential author—at least as far as the unregulated use of essential oils by presumably uninformed laypeople is concerned.

Availability of Valnet's and Tisserand's books to a broader public outside the francophone world must be credited with making aromatherapy a household word. The way aromatherapy was perceived was gradually changing. It became to be seen as an intriguing semimedical modality that allowed the layperson to attempt self-therapy for many common ailments. But along with the growing popularity of aromatherapy, other different and diverse interpretations have since developed—some rather esoteric, others concentrating on the olfactory aspect.

In retrospect, it appears that it was in fact the popularity of aromatherapy that spawned the broadening commercial and scientific interests in the effects of fragrance and olfaction. Because commercial exploitation of the medical use of essential oils is legally restricted or completely prohibited in many Western societies, the fragrance aspect of the aromatherapy phenomenon received the lion's share of commercial interest. It steered clear of potential conflict with existing regulations. After 1980, the aro-

Figure 1.1: Stepping stones in the development of aromatherapy

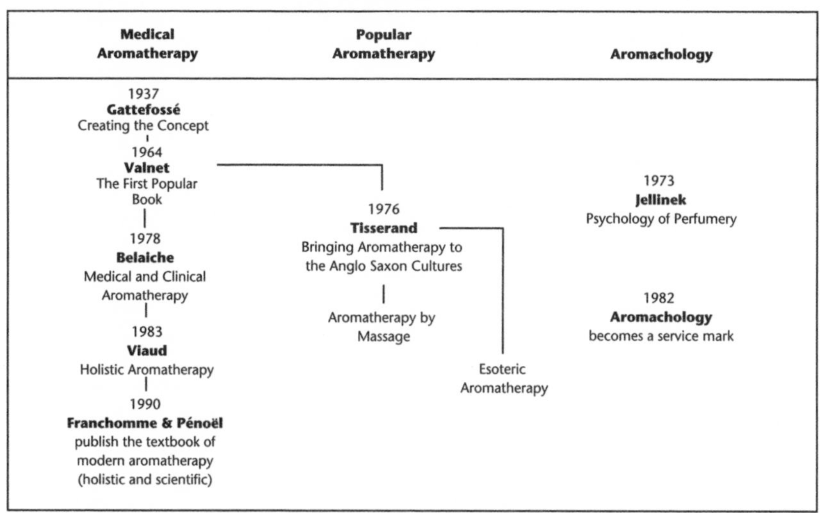

matherapy phenomenon diversified into four basic avenues: medical and holistic-medical aromatherapy as practiced in France, popular and esoteric aromatherapy as found in publications in most Western societies, aromatherapy applied during massage as practiced mainly in Great Britain, and the scientific study of fragrance as encouraged by the Fragrance Research Fund, the latter avenue more precisely referred to as *aroma-chology*. A summary of cornerstones of these developments is given in Figure 1.

Medical aromatherapy

The treatment of infections with essential oils was extensively researched by Paul Belaiche.[6] This work, published in 1979, is still unique. It combines extensive in-vitro research on the antimicrobial effects of essential oils with their corresponding clinical application. The French aromatherapy tradition continued with the publication in 1990 of *L'aromathérapie exactement*, by Pierre Franchomme and Daniel Pénoël, the current textbook of medical aromatherapy.[7] It combines modern scientific arguments with a clearly holistic orientation, and seeks to understand the effects of essential oils based on the synergistic pharmacology of all of their constituents. The bias of the authors is that unaltered essential oils are always superior to synthetic, semisynthetic, or so-called nature identical substances. They consider genuine essential oils superior despite (or because) they are subject to a natural variation of their composition brought about by differing distillation processes or variation of climate or similar factors. (See page XX.) Unique stereochemical or enantiomeric proportions and the influence of trace substances are seen as two identifiable reasons for this superiority because they represent keys to a biological compatibility—between humans and oils—that is not found with synthetic substances. The therapeutic value of aromatherapy is based on the biological effects of genuine (unaltered) and authentic (from only one, clearly identified species) essential oils.[8] The intrinsic composition and qualities of synthetics—despite misleading terms such as "nature identical"—is not the same. Appreciating this difference led to modest commercial responses. Smaller or family-owned operations began producing essential oils for the needs of the aromatherapy market, while established large-scale manufacturers and/or brokers often remained unimpressed by the relatively minute volumes involved.

Robert Tisserand's book *The Art of Aromatherapy* soon drew a wider audience to the concepts of aromatherapy in English- and German-speaking societies, and a gradual expansion of aromatherapy literature ensued. Most of the early literature following the publication of Tisserand's book originated in Great Britain and was authored by laywomen. In the early eighties, at the dawn of the rising popularity of aromatherapy, information was so scarce that an aromatherapy enthusiast would often purchase every book on the subject that became available. But soon the topic had garnered such momentum that the number of published titles increased sharply. Keeping track of all of them became virtually impossible. This sharp increase in interest can be attributed to a large degree to the popular style of Tisserand's *The Art of Aromatherapy*, which made the concepts of aromatherapy accessible to everyone and removed it from its isolation as an appendix to medical academia. Massage therapists and laypeople entered the field in growing numbers and quickly turned it into an economic reality.

The nonacademic character of aromatherapy in England is probably a main reason why it is confronted with a certain antagonism from the conventional medical establishment. The results of this antagonism are obvious in the whole body of British aromatherapy literature. An author's desire to communicate the realm of possible healing with aromatherapy collides with the fear of being penalized by the conventional system if that system's turf is invaded. A disenchanting stream of disclaimers and rampant self-censorship (constantly telling the reader never to do this and never to do that) are the hallmarks of commercially inspired confusion of regulations and truths.

While the British developments are equated by many with the development of aromatherapy in general, sometimes sharp differences exist in the course aromatherapy has taken in different regions and cultures. An exploration of the factors that contributed to these differences is as entertaining as it is enlightening. The direction aromatherapy took in France remained scientific and medical, yet ultimately alternative. Germany developed its own rather esoteric aromatherapy scene, and Australia had its own British-influenced brand of the new therapy. But it was England where aromatherapy flourished as a form of massage therapy and ultimately was characterized as a complementary modality.[9]

The striking differences between the French and British approaches are explained by taking a look at who turned to this modality. In France, aromatherapy was first propagated by medical doctors, as evidenced by the above-mentioned three-volume aromatherapy textbook of Paul Belaiche and Franchomme and Pénoël's *L'aromathérapie exactement*. The fact that the original texts in France were authored by doctors led to a substantial integration of aromatherapy into conventional medicine.

It is ironic that the ability of the medical system to appreciate the value of aromatherapy can be so distinctly different in two neighboring societies. What is accepted by doctors in some countries is marginalized in others, especially in Great Britain and the United States, which suggests that issues of status, and the protection of economic monopolies, are thoroughly muddled with what is officially disseminated as objective and scientific rigor.

The pattern of popular appreciation of aromatherapy and consequent (perceived) hostility of the medical system repeated itself in the United States a few years later. Many small businesses were started with little or no grasp of regulatory realities, but took their cues from highly dominant British aromatherapy influences. FDA became a three-letter acronym that made the typical upstart aromatherapy entrepreneur rife with irrational angst. Not angering the medical profession is still a prominent objective in U.S./English aromatherapy literature, as preemptive self-censorship continues unabated. The apparent insecurity is obvious in the choice of language. Many authors have taken to a typical aromatherapy phraseology where every statement is immediately qualified or made conditional: "Oil of [insert any name] may be [or is said to be] helpful for [enter any condition]" became the dominant phrase of aromatherapy writing. Whether threats by regulatory agencies and hostility from the medical system in the United States and in Great Britain were only perceived or real, they effectively prohibited the development of medical aromatherapy as it is at least tolerated in France and those countries where large corporations cannot directly influence the legislative process.

The commercialization of aromatherapy

Nonetheless, the magnetism of aromatherapy attracted an increasing number of followers, and commercialization of its less controversial aspects became the preferred and safest conduit for satisfying the related desires. This is reflected in many lavishly illustrated coffee-table volumes with intriguing and sensuous pictures of exotic botanicals and lithe bodies. What precious little text there is, floating on four-color photographs, is overshadowed by the splendor of the graphic design. "Information" contained in these books is typically a variation of recipes for blending more or less the same commercially available essential oils into concoctions of esoteric, spiritual, or even practical allure. Fragrant solutions, ranging from "goddess" blends with astrological significance to blends that promise to influence fertility and inspiration are mainly directed towards women's spiritual needs. But although many of these alluring books are born out of transparent motive and exploitative calculation, they are also evidence that an awareness of the connection between aroma, consciousness, and the spiritual dimension is growing.

Looking at these contemporary aromatherapy books, one might gain the impression that aromatherapy evolved directly from ancient Egypt into the body shops of the world. But this form of catchy marketing is at best half true, as it equates aromatherapy with ancient practice. Yet today's aromatherapy is distinctly different from the general use of aromatic plants throughout history. "Aromatherapy" as the term is used today originated (by Réné-Maurice Gattefossé) in the first half of the twentieth century in the spirit of scientific exploration. Before World War II, the exploration of essential oils drew as much scientific interest as the exploration of other drugs. Identifying the components of natural essential oils was one of the big tasks and, ultimately, successes of chemistry. The development of chemistry owes a great deal to essential oil research; indeed, Nobel prizes were awarded to Otto Wallach and Adolf von Baeyer, two of the most outstanding researchers in the field, for their contributions in uncovering the secrets of essential oils. Their stories are fascinating, and until now have not been included in aromatherapy lore (see page 88). From this same period date the first attempts to classify essential oils according to the chemistry of their components—a concept that permeates the theory and practice of French medical aromatherapy even today.

Indeed, it is in the last decade of the twentieth century where aromatherapy has received its most emphatic welcome in the Western industrialized societies, all of which have—to varying degrees—tied their medical systems to the scientific model.

Because aromatherapy finds its strongest popular base in those countries where it is most marginalized by official medicine, I suspect that it evolved as a response to that system. It is well known that the cost of bringing new drugs to market is extremely high and is an option that is in reality only available to the huge corporations.[10]

It is much less well known that corporate capital has also taken over hospitals almost completely.[11] The stage is set. On one side is a pharmaceutical and HMO industry grossing about a trillion dollars per year in the United States alone. Corporate power convinces almost every citizen that drugs and medical procedures are the most effective, reasonable, and responsible means to cure diseases. On the other side there are human beings who despite lifelong conditioning—often more realistically called indoctrination—opt to choose other routes of healing. It may be impossible to provide a figure on what percentage of the population staunchly believes in conventional medicine and what proportion is moving towards alternatives. But it is possible to identify the trend, as one third of all visits to a health practitioner in the United States at this time are paid to providers of alternative therapies.

Taking control

What brings people to aromatherapy? What exactly is it that stimulates many mothers to try and care for their children with natural means, often with aromatherapy? What is it that makes some people take to aromatherapy immediately? How is aromatherapy different from conventional medicine? And how is aromatherapy different from other alternative modalities?

The answers to these questions begin with the realization that aromatherapy is a dynamic process, not a static system of prescribing remedies. Aromatherapy can initiate the first steps on a journey that will ultimately lead to becoming master of one's own health. At the start of the journey, an individual may be firmly rooted in the conventional way of looking at health and disease. In this position, one typically has strong beliefs in the infectious, genetic, environmental, nature of disease. Disease is most likely seen as the consequence of a logically identifiable cause, very often pathogenic bacteria, but also as a consequence of certain dietary mistakes or other factors connected to lifestyle. The existence of somatic factors, such as stress or emotional influences, is usually accepted in general terms but mostly ruled out to be of relevance in the specific symptoms. If disease strikes, it is considered an arbitrary event brought on by a material cause. Generally, responsibility is turned over to the medical expert whose recommendations are followed and whose prescriptions are taken. This is one possible view of health and disease, and many individuals who live by this concept despite debilitating dependency on thirty pills every day as well as numerous surgeries lead full and productive lives.

This form of medicine *can* work; those who look for alternatives are not necessarily driven by blatant failures of the old system but by changing concepts of health, varying degrees of skepticism toward the policies of mainstream medical commerce, and possibly a concern about the overall direction of human life on this planet.

On the other side of the spectrum are individuals who realize that health can also be maintained through prudent exercise of personal abilities and responsibility, without humiliating dependence on the current medical system. Much of what is passed off as necessary by the conventional system is really just a marketing ploy. Finding balance with the help of time-tested modalities is found to be a significantly less expensive way to maintain health.

One of the special qualities of aromatherapy is that it has the power, through its immediacy (interaction with many of the mind/body regulating circuits, discussed in Chapter 6), to start the transformation from dependence to independence. Aromatherapy will not sustain the whole transformation. As individuals become more experienced, typically other modalities such as acupuncture and TCM (traditional Chinese medicine) are integrated. But aromatherapy is a unique initial stimulant, which offers many effective methods for the prevention and cure of infections as well as the prevention of diseases resulting from unavoidable imbalances of urban life. How can that be? Is this too good to be true?

Some of the answers are in this book

In Chapter 2, I'll explain that revitalizing olfactory abilities and instilling a renewed appreciation for natural scents, ranging from those of flowers, forest, and ocean to those naturally present on human bodies, strengthens individual identity under assault from the loss of odor mandated by clean-shaven, corporate societies. Olfactory traits of an individual and immune response are programmed in an identical set of genes. That strengthening olfactory identity would therefore strengthen defensive mechanisms seems logical.

Chapter 3 points out that the substances of aromatherapy, essential oils, are distinguished by their molecular makeup. Every single molecule found in essential oils (or at least its precursor before steam distillation) has been a part of the evolutionary development of life. The tolerability, compatibility, and effectiveness of these molecules has developed over hundreds of millions of years and proven itself by the survival of those organisms that produce them. As life unfolded, aroma molecules were present at every stage of development and have consequently become part and parcel of many biological processes. They interact harmoniously with all biological systems at once, with the combined effect being highly favorable. Synthetics, to the contrary, have not proven themselves on any substantial timescale, and the resulting disasters—when approval processes were simply not capable of predicting even short-term effects—are horrid legacy to this.

Nonetheless, the argument has been made that assumptions about the generally biocompatible nature of essential oils are patently unsubstantiated because throughout evolution, plants—and also other organisms—have developed both benign and highly toxic substances. According to the conventional standpoint, all substances have to be considered potentially harmful until declared safe by scientific assessment. This reasoning is obviously based on a physicalist worldview according to which the universe consists of dead matter floating around in space. Yet recently a new class of genes has been discovered that predetermine the spectrum of variance available to evolution. Accordingly, the range of compounds a plant can produce is not unlimited but will follow a clear pattern and remain within specific boundaries. Arguments that the benign or toxic character of natural substances is totally arbitrary are mute in light of these new findings.

The range of secondary plant substances that is indeed toxic is well known to humanity and it is very unlikely that an aromatherapy aficionado will unwittingly encounter an entirely new class of unexpected killer molecules in essential oils.

In plants we always encounter a complex set of components that exert their effects on the human body in highly controlled ways, in which one substance will act to stimulate and another to calm down. (This is discussed in greater detail in Chapter 4.) The net effect is positive, as this system can be seen as having built-in feedback loops: if one action is too strong, the counteracting substance is right there for the body to use. Nature recognizes limits. The complex chemical composition of plant drugs is one expression of that. In pharmacology, complex mixtures of plant substances are too unyielding and too hard to standardize, and one might also suspect too hard to be monopolized. Consequently, synthetic drugs often are inspired by molecular concepts found in nature. But in order to make them of use to the system, presumed active components are first isolated from the molecular environment present in the plant and then chemically altered, ostensibly to make them more effective but also to make them patentable and thus useful for the profit motive.

What happens when the feedback loops—originally present in the whole mixture of plant substances—are eliminated in the quest for higher effectiveness is illustrated graphically with the example of illegal drugs. Andean native peoples have chewed coca leaves since prehistory and have consequently become competent in handling this natural drug. This is in stark contrast to the sociopathic destruction following isolation and subsequent modification of the cocaine molecule that turn the substance into crack. A similar parallel can be drawn between the use of poppy plants and the destruction associated with heroin.

Certain elements of the above ideas have scientific corroboration, but to prove these concepts as a whole and scientifically is practically impossible. Admittedly, these concepts are more easily grasped philosophically with vitalist arguments that acknowledge the botanical core of medicine.[12]

In Chapter 5, we will see that no matter how much we would like to con ourselves into thinking otherwise, disastrous effects are not limited to illegal drugs. The profit motive and a supporting cast of economically dependent scientists and corporate lobbyists have pushed dubious drugs through the approval process, from which more Americans have died than from the Vietnam war. All of this has been foreseen by Ivan Illich in his book *Medical Nemesis*.[13] He reasons that in medicine the ultimate hubris of playing God will bring about the wrath of the gods, making medicine the leading cause of disease. There are countless ways in which the current system of science in the employ of commerce is trying to obscure this reality by conditioning everyone in the Western world to believe that only medicines developed by research, requiring high technology and great expense somewhere along their production process, can be considered truly effective and desirable. This has ensured that control over health care has gone entirely to big capital. Money will always follow the profit motive, as has been evidenced lately by the increasingly shameless maneuvers of HMOs. The issue at hand is whether profit motive and free-market dogma really are the best concepts to base health care on. After all, I would not expect the large pharmaceutical organizations to come up with an inexpensive cure even if it was easily available. Science and commerce combine to monopolize the market as well as our perceptions about healing.

Most of the time these days, science articulates itself in a rather unobjective (unscientific) and political manner to intimidate people who in following their instincts prefer natural means and reject some of the cures science has cooked up for us. (This idea is discussed in greater detail in Chapter 6.) This is observed when the *New England Journal of Medicine* presents "objective" editorials but hides the identity of their authors who in fact are partisan industry representatives. [14]

Every once in a while there are exceptions to the rule and science is actually employed to probe into the physiological effects of essential oils. This can produce rather stunning results, such as the demonstration of antiviral or antitumor activity for common essential-oil components. Aromatherapy has benefited greatly from a few precious scientific contributions. The best seems yet to come as the complex interactions between essential-oil components and the various receptor systems of the body become better understood.

In Chapter 7, we will see that the current economic system has produced enormous amounts of suffering and has placed society in an advanced state of disintegration, including environmental diseases, rampant depression, and destitute inner cities. The industrial medical complex is part and parcel of this economic system and the cures it has to offer for the most pressing problems (those mentioned above as well as heart disease, arthritis, cancer, and AIDS) are ridiculously ineffective despite the staggering amounts of money the system charges society for its services. It is only a matter of time until there is a change in perception about the exorbitant cost of the medical system. The one thousand billion dollars spent are perceived as suffocating, but they also represent an enormous market. It will be argued that alternative health will become the largest economic sector. Modalities such as aromatherapy, which acknowledge the phenomena of the soul, will be vastly more successful in treating the real problems of our times than conventional medicine. Medicine as it stands is part of the problem, therefore it can do very little for its solution. Once a way for acceptable deregulation of health care is accepted, the dam will break and alternative modalities will gain market share explosively.

As pointed out earlier, aromatherapy currently means different things to different people. This is not surprising considering that it maneuvers in the transition zone from one paradigm to another. Trying to gain acceptance for aromatherapy by the conventional system, that is, hoping that doctors would start to implement it if there only was more scientific documentation, is counterproductive. It ignores the fact that scientific procedures have long lost their independence and serve mainly to perpetuate the economic status quo. Establishing the aromatherapist as a new expert who dispenses this new therapy to laypeople perceived as ignorant and not able to take responsibility for their own health repeats one of the worst traits of conventional medicine.

Chapter 8 describes how to overcome the difficulties of moving from a mechanistic to a vitalistic manner of health care, and Chapter 9 lays out the concepts for a new way to approach self-medication and self-care, acknowledging how aromatherapy excels through simplicity.

Chapter 10 points out that aromatherapy contributes to the realization of health what no material science can—it accepts and integrates phenomena of the soul. Essential oil molecules are so intricately involved with the chemistry of life that their interactions with an organism are much too numerous to be even approximated by scientific inquiry. They interact with physical systems via receptors, they play important roles in the psychosomatic network, and through olfaction they interact with emotional centers. Through the combined effect of all of the above, they create powerful imprints on our consciousness. Gaining insight into the workings of essential oils triggers constructive questions about the whole interlocking system of life on this planet. The aromatherapy experience is far from irrational; it leaves the known systems of physics, chemistry, and biology intact. It is this respect for the creation inherent in aromatherapy that motivates those who turn to aromatherapy. For those choosing to do so, a higher order is squarely visible in the many ways essential oils interact with organisms. Fragrance has always transcended the material planes of consciousness (science) and communicated directly with those of the soul (the psycho-social plane). While aromatherapy accepts a hierarchical order of the planes of consciousness, it does not commit the fatal mistake of trying to explain the psycho-social and the spiritual plane of consciousness with the means of the lower material plane. Aromatherapy does not mandate a spiritual belief system, but it is practically self-evident that catching a glimpse of the interdependence of all life will make the concept of a higher order very appealing. As such, aromatherapy has in it the spiritual element that American Indians have always recognized in plants. As such, aromatherapy has the ingredient of healing that is missing the most in the materialistic modalities.

Chapter 11 introduces the manner in which essential-oil molecules are tied to many other important biological molecules by their common biosynthesis. Factors unique to the natural composition of essential oils are presented, such as the presence of trace components of extremely high odor impact. A brief summary of safety is given and the popular notion of the superior safety of natural substances is explored.

Chapter 12 presents a chemical classification of the components occurring in essential oils and discusses the properties of essential oils that result from the synergistic actions between the most important main components of a given oil.

Chapter 13 gives application methods for essential oils that are unique to aromatherapy and not influenced by traditional thought. Aromatherapy treatment regimens are presented for a variety of ailments, with a concentration on those that work particularly well and have not yet been extensively described in the literature.

Aromatherapy's renaissance

It is easy to speculate that this willing embrace of a modality like aromatherapy is a reaction to the loss of nature. Many of us possess a very deep-seated intuition that not every illness and every ill can be healed with more technology and more pharmacology. Perhaps the belief that more research will solve practically any medical problem represents the ultimate hubris.

There is probably a strong intuition that maintaining balance with the world we live in is a more effective approach to the maintenance of good health than the warlike concepts of conventional medicine. Yet, because these aggressive principles are the most widely accepted and internalized in the Western industrial societies, there is a deeper desire for an antidote. In Mediterranean and Latin societies, where the general use of herbs and natural medicine to maintain balance and health have never been banished as vigorously as in Anglo-Saxon and especially North American societies, this desire is still present. The need to revitalize plant medicine and aroma is not as strong in these societies because it was never lost to begin with. Nor is there any need in the countries and societies of the developing world, where the traditional healing systems have never given up on plant medicine.

"The boof is not unattractive, yet when I test it,
I have somehow the feeling that I am
smelling the sinister vapors of fascism.
—Tom Robbins, *Jitterbug Perfume*

TWO

Odor Is Identity

Our sense of smell, once a vital and essential tool for survival, lost all its significance in the transition from natural to more industrialized and high-tech lifestyles. It is quite likely that losing our appreciation for natural fragrances is merely the most obvious symptom, that we have also lost other faculties inherent in a natural lifestyle. Marginalizing our sense of smell had a strong impact on different aspects of human life, from the cultural to the spiritual and from mating choices to immune response. A subconscious desire to regain what was lost is a driving force of the surging popularity of the aroma field.

The work of Paolo Rovesti

Paolo Rovesti studied the effects of fragrances on the psyche long before current interest in aromatherapy made it a popular topic.[1] Traveling around the globe, he researched the role of fragrance in past cultures, such as the many ways fragrance was integrated into spiritual, magical, and social rituals. To understand what the elimination of fragrance in our techno-culture means, we shall follow some of Rovesti's musings. He noted that rising anosmia among individuals in highly civilized societies was well documented, and he considered the decreased ability to perceive odor to be the direct consequence of emotional and nervous stress associated with urban living. He blamed "...the hugely successful concept of installing apparatuses satisfying the needs of the other senses, especially of sight and hearing..." for audio and visual sensation overload. Existing indoors, in subways, and in office towers makes a breeze of fresh air a rarity. By the late sixties, Rovesti had observed the particular intensity and uniformity with which "consumer goods in Japan and in U.S. drug stores are perfumed with synthetic fragrances."

It appears that Rovesti's predictions about the cultural consequences of a denial of smell, coupled with a merciless dominance of sight and hearing, have been exceeded by reality. As we will see, odor, especially personal body odor as we emanate it and as we perceive it, is highly individual. It is an important part of who we are. According to Rovesti, the suppression of scent has robbed individuals of their identity, leaving them open to be manipulated by assaults on the senses of sight and hearing, molding individuals into faceless masses.[2]

Consequences of the denial of smell

An example comes from our image and sound factories, also known as the movie industry. Hollywood films are discussed by exceedingly large segments of society as if they were cultural events or attempts at art. Before entertainment became an industrially identified need, a writer or a director normally aimed at expressing something in an artistic fashion. But the artists' desire to express has given way to the drive for success, measured in sales. We consider those sports, musical, or movie stars "successful" who generate the highest sales, surrendering our own judgment and instincts to mass opinion. If a movie breaks a box-office record it must somehow be worthy and good.

Today's Hollywood movies are, first and foremost, corporate

products with the singular goal to create box-office sensations and make money. Success is no longer measured by mastery of artistic expression, but by finding the broadest common denominator and selling more than the competition. It is well known that these common denominators are found by appealing to the lowest human instincts. It is not so obvious that the subsequent decline in human behavior is a privilege of the manipulated senses of sight and hearing. There are people who say that seeing blood and guts splattered on a movie screen constitutes entertainment. Sick as it sounds, that notion would vanish in a second if they also had to smell it.

This type of success, where half of the population watches an entertainment product all on the same weekend, would not too long ago have been viewed quite differently. Manipulating large numbers of people into behaving the same way was considered a manifestation of fascism. For Etruscan kings and subsequently in the Rome of antiquity, a homogeneous bundle of sticks, equally long and wide, was the ruler's symbol of power over his subjects. These bundles of identical sticks were called *fasci*.

Calling the phenomenon of movie mania a variation of fascism will strike many as an exaggeration. Aren't those movie-goers watching these movies out of their own will? Weren't people *forced* into submission by fascist regimes? This is true. The fact remains, millions of people *are* behaving in the same way. What has changed is not the desire to rule, control, and manipulate but the means of coercion. This loss of individuality in mass-market society has evolved conspicuously parallel to the sense of smell becoming almost irrelevant.

The eradication of natural odor plays a enormous role in transforming a large number of individuals into a homogeneous mass of people with identical preferences, behavior, and feelings. The language that perpetuates this uniformity identifies the hidden instigators of this process. In Orwellian fashion, one way to control thoughts and feelings is to reverse meanings. An expression that at one point meant one thing implies something entirely different in the new streamlined reality. "Adult"means porn. "Conservative" means to favor relentless exploitation, and "Just Do It" somehow stands for overpriced shoes. Polluting oil companies laud their environmental record. Pesticide manufacturers genetically manipulate seeds in the name of feeding the hungry. It is probably not too far-fetched to conclude that any public announcement by a large corporation means the opposite of what is said on the surface. Love is hate, peace is war, and, most importantly, ignorance is wisdom.

Toward uniform flavors and fragrances

These examples demonstrate to what extent creation of uniformity is possible by manipulating the senses of sight and hearing. What we see and hear can be almost fully manipulated by technological culture. The sense of smell, in evolutionary terms, resides in a much more ancient area of the brain and is more archaic. Biologically, the sense of smell is intimately connected with our vital instincts and safeguarded against manipulation—to *some* degree, but not completely.

It is also possible to manipulate the senses of smell and taste into accepting uniformity, which a return to the movie-craze metaphor can illustrate. Many who watch these "movies of the moment" will also eat Big Macs, but at least they know they are not consuming a work of art. But there are untiring efforts by the big food conglomerates to do to taste and smell what has already been accomplished in the sight and hearing realm. A telling statement by a CEO of a flavor and fragrance corporation illustrates this:

> The trend to health foods, already well begun here, will spread. Removal of the culprits—fat, calories, sugar, salt, cholesterol, all taste good—must be compensated for with flavor replacements. We call them flavor systems since they do not provide merely the flavor, but a number of other aspects required for the taste experience—mouthfeel, moisture content, browning effect, and so forth. Prepared foods for vegetarians and others require savory flavors (such as meat, cheese, chicken) to make them more palatable. Low-fat yogurt and low-fat cheese, nonalcoholic wines and beers, flavored teas, flavors

> for sugarless desserts, dairy products and cereals are some other areas with new flavor demands...Flavored mineral waters and "New Age" beverages which contain fruit juices and high impact flavors are now reaching Europe also...and those who believe Europeans will not succumb to adventuresome taste experiences may be making a critical marketing mistake.[3]

The research effort going into producing these sensations is enormous, and reflects the mind-set that we will encounter over and over, namely that with enough science in the name of commerce man can actually improve on nature. In Illich's words this is hubris. The diseases that follow the prolonged consumption of these entirely untested aroma mixtures are the nemesis that follows.[4] In a sinister way, it is even reflected in the jargon in which flavor corporations describe the products with which they "enhance" our lives. WONF is a recognized acronym and stands for "with other natural flavors." "Natural," in this context, means that the original starting material had to be natural but a number of alterations via chemical modification of this material are accepted.

> Today's state-of-the-art natural WONF formulations result in products that more closely resemble the taste found in nature and are much more effective in food products than traditional compositions, especially when they are adequately functionalized. These strawberry, cherry and peach formulas are composed mostly of discreet isolates...and look more like a list of components found in the analysis of a natural extract. Such compounds find use in fortification of juiced-based flavors, improving both the overall taste and the in-use strength of the WONFs.[5]

Thus it has to be conceded that corporate efforts to create uniform mass consciousness succeed even in the areas of flavor, slyly accomplished again by cleverly implying a given product will enhance a consumer's individuality but really selling a mass-produced, one-dimensional flavor product.[6] The principle works in almost every area of modern civilized life but is exemplified by the relation the media has with the public. The media does what the word says—they mediate people. The concept was originated by none other than Napoleon. It means giving a small, overrun prince or sovereign the illusion of power by allowing him to nominally keep his title while really governing his fiefdom on remote control from Paris. In Napoleon's word he was mediated, much better-sounding than "useful idiot."Today this goal, to mediate, has become the main purpose of the media: to maintain an illusion of freedom and individuality while in reality brainwashing everyone into becoming mindless consumers. We keep on purchasing more useless, plastic goods. One has to wonder how the advertisements of mass-market products do it—somehow they can sell twenty million ordinary suitcases with two "magical" letters on it and still allow the purchaser to believe that the product is a supreme expression of exclusivity.

Because it is globalization that has allowed corporate strategists to exercise their power in an increasingly overt way, one might ask, in the tradition of Rovesti, whether the many inhumane consequences of globalization also have an odor element. And they do! Large segments of the workforce have been effectively manipulated to believe that they are interchangeable and need to compete with cheap labor in far-away countries. This reflects the lack of identity and conversely the high degree of uniformity encountered in the artificial fragrances favored in today's corporate world. Underarm hair, which is responsible for a person's individual odor profile, is frowned upon. This is especially true for women, whose identity and individuality has to remain banished from the male domain of coldly exercising corporate power. Female compassion and underarm hair would be unruly. To be a good mid-level corporate agent one is first deodorized and then wrapped in the most prevalent fragrances the temples of consumerism have to offer. Perfumes encountered in airports, discotheques, and other "happening" places of the industrial world manifest this uniformity. From Singapore to Los Angeles, New York to Johannesburg, the "in" spots reek of artificial fruit notes similar to those found in the Day-Glo-colored candies favored by the youngest members of society.

Fragrance in literature

As manipulation of fragrance became a cofactor in eliminating individuality, the ritual uses of fragrance, once common in all cultures, died out completely and for quite some time almost no one seemed to miss it. Yet only a hundred years ago, the use of aromatic plants was still a big part of cultural life. A beautiful example is Gabriel Garcia Marquez's description of Dr. Urbino Juvenal, eminent physician in a coastal Caribbean town in the late nineteenth century:

> He arose at the crack of dawn, when he began to take his secret medicines: potassium bromide to raise his spirits, salicylates for the ache in his bones when it rained, ergosterol drops for vertigo, belladonna for sound sleep. He took something every hour, always in secret, because in his long life as a doctor and teacher he had always opposed prescribing palliatives for old age: it was easier for him to bear other peoples' pain than his own. In his pocket he always carried a little pad of camphor that he inhaled deeply when no one was watching to calm his fear of so many medications mixed together.[7]

The association of fragrances with romantic and philosophical aspects of life, common in the literature of the nineteenth and early twentieth century, has disappeared almost completely. Notable exceptions are two novels dealing specifically with smell: *Perfume* and *Jitterbug Perfume*.[8] The use of fragrance or essential oils in the context of magic became extinct not only because the importance of fragrance diminished, but because, in the scientific age, there is no such thing as magic. Interesting though that we do accept the concept of magic in a certain sense when connected to the dominant senses of sight and hearing as special effects in movies.[9]

How important the sense of smell must have been in more natural living societies is illustrated by experiments Rovesti performed repeatedly. Individuals in indigenous societies he visited were able to identify other men and women solely by scent while Rovesti and his fellow travelers were unable to do the same.

Body odor: the facts

Rovesti's observation that individuals have a distinct, specific odor—a chemical signature—could later be verified by controlled experiments. Ongoing studies at The Monell Institute of Taste and Smell Research in Philadelphia have revealed that the olfactory system can recognize genetic differences in the immune system. Humans are also individuals immunologically: body odor and immune system are linked in all mammals. Dr. Lewis Thomas, a former chairman of Monell, took his original clue from observing that both olfactory and immune systems were able to identify aspects of individuality. Noting that dogs were able to track the scent of a specific human across a field containing numerous other human odors, he concluded that each individual must also have a distinctive odor and that the olfactory system is capable of discriminating these odors from one another.

Similarly, the immune system has the ability to distinguish self from other, a fundamental property of individual recognition. To a large extent, this ability is linked to a set of more than fifty genes, known as the major histocompatibility complex (MHC). Genes in the MHC are critical to many aspects of immune function. Virtually every individual, with the exception of identical twins, has a unique MHC due to the extreme diversity of MHC genes. The immune system will generally attack any cell with a foreign MHC.[10] It was therefore hypothesized that the immune and olfactory systems were related and that the immune-regulating MHC genes also establish controlled olfactory uniqueness.

In experiments with mice, males preferred to mate with females possessing MHC genes different from their own, which leads to reduced inbreeding and enhanced genetic diversity. It was also possible to show that mating preference is determined by olfactory cues. Mice can distinguish between the odors of urine of other mice that differ only in their MHC. This shows that the MHC genes are linked to the makeup of individual odor. MHC-determined odors (now termed "odor types") can be altered by varying only a single gene within the MHC.

That odor types play a role in human communication and behavior has been a basic notion of every culture. Monell research suggests that odor cues conveyed through sweat, saliva, or mother's milk are strongly influenced by diet and environment, but most dramatically by genetic factors. It has also been established that human fetuses have distinct odor types and that smell serves as the first means of bonding between mother and newborn child.

Underarm odor is generated from the secretions of the apocrine glands, which are mainly located on the scalp, the cheeks, the underarms, the anogenital areas, and the areola of the nipples. Microorganisms residing on underarm hair chemically alter the original secretions to give the underarms their typical odor profile. The molecules originally secreted and the resulting odorants are closely related to the steroidal sex hormone testosterone. Two of the main steroidal substances contributing to axillary odor are androstenone, with a typical urinous odor, and androstenol, which has a musky odor. Steroids are products of the same biochemical assembly line in the cell as the terpene molecules of essential oils; they are both components of the basic chemistry of human instincts.[11]

Table 2.1: Important Odorants in Axillary Odor

Odorant	**Fragrance**
Androstenone	urinous
Androstenol	musky
(E)-3-Methyl-hex-2-enoic acid	axillary
4-Ethyl-heptanoic acid	hircine
Isovaleric acid	sweaty

The scientific understanding of body odor took a big leap when it became obvious that not only steroid molecules but also unique, unsaturated fatty acids contribute to axillary odor. In the summer of 1990 a flurry of headlines announced a new breakthrough in the research of underarm odor chemistry: "Scientists find chemical clue to body odor," (*New York Times*, August 1990); "Key ingredient in armpit odor sniffed out," (*Washington Post*, August 1990); "Scientist sniffs out culprit in damp case," (*Herald Tribune*, August 1990); "Stink tank scientists report body odor breakthrough," (*Japan Times*, August 1990). These headlines all referred to the new work at the Monell Center that showed that isovaleric acid (sweaty-foot odor), 3-Methylhex-2-enoic acid (axillary sweat odor), 4 Ethylheptanoic acid (goat odor, hirsutine), and a host of other similar components contributed strongly to axillary odor.

It is now understood that every person produces his or her unique mix of these and other odoriferous compounds, which make up a person's individual scent. In addition, there are gender-specific "labels": men secrete more odorant and have more dermal bacteria than women, which explains the stronger and more pungent odors typically encountered in males. Men also excrete larger quantities of steroids, resulting in higher concentrations of androstenone and androstenol. Interestingly, these steroids are also found in the plant world: in truffles and in celery.

The forgotten magic of body odor

Another key to understanding the complexity of these phenomena was found when it was observed that some individuals were anosmic to certain chemicals in the axillary mix, and that other individuals were anosmic to two or more of these chemicals. This means that everybody has his or her unique perception of another person's axillary odor. For example, individual A may be anosmic to androstenone and, consequently, would not smell the urinous component in someone's body odor. Individual B may be anosmic to androstenone and to 3-Methylhex-2-enoic acid and, consequently, have an odor impression quite different from someone able to smell all the substances present. From the variety of components contributing to body odor to the many ways our individual mix of anosmias (or their absence) affects our fragrance perceptions, there is almost an infinite number of odor combinations possible. This is a major reason why matters of body odor are so uniquely personal.[12]

The individual traits of body odor and olfaction are embedded in cultural aspects of fragrance recognition and preference. Taking into account that these odorants can influence reproductive parameters (such as harmonized menstrual cycles between cohabitating women) or have, to some degree, pheromonal character, it is clear that many varied and complex messages may be processed by this system at any time. It appears that these messages may have a much deeper influence on human life and behavior than we are ready to concede. Not surprisingly, preindustrial societies approach this phenomenon with the metaphors of magic. In healing rituals of certain tribes, the female or male healer takes sweat from his or her own armpit and places it on the ill person. Traditional south sea islanders wear tufts of sweet-smelling plants near their axilla, giving them a scent that combines their own odor with plant odor. This is reminiscent of traditional Western perfumery, in which the malodors of the anogenital orifices, reminiscent of sex, are combined with pleasant odors such as floral and/or stimulants to create pleasant erogenous complexes.

"Life has helped me cure diseases that other doctors cause with their medicines."
—Gabriel Garcia Marquez, *Of Love and Other Demons*

THREE

Evolution and Pesto

Why do we pick snails off of our basil plants? Answer: Because we want to harvest healthy bunches of basil to make pesto or other culinary delights. While we may consider this to be good gardening practice, we are probably not aware that we are tipping the evolutionary scale in favor of the survival of one species over another. We help the basil plant because of its culinary qualities. This practice is not limited to potted basil plants in backyards, it is repeated on a fairly large industrial scale. Sizable amounts of basil oil are used in the food-processing industry and to a lesser degree in the perfume industry.

In aromatherapy, basil holds a special position. There is extreme diversity within the species and subspecies of basil, which display different chemical compositions and, consequently, different properties. A survey of the available literature shows that it is nearly impossible to find an ailment for which basil would not at least be somewhat helpful, from restoring movement to paralyzed limbs to its effectiveness against the polio virus. Even if not every author's praise of basil's healing qualities can be a hundred percent verified, it is true that this oil in particular and essential oils in general have an astonishingly broad range of preventive and healing properties. Why is this so?

Biocompatibility, tolerability, and effectiveness of the natural chemical compounds that comprise essential oils are a result of hundreds of millions of years of biochemical trial and error called evolution. Essential oil components are produced in the cell following a biosynthetic pathway, which existed in the first life forms on the planet.[1] Does this have any relevance for holistic aromatherapy, or for the holistic approach in general? A very short history of aromatic substances could shed some light on this question.

A brief history of aromatic plant substances

Somewhere between four and two billion years ago, life began with single-celled organisms. These simple cells were perfectly designed to manufacture, among many other molecules, terpenes, the main constituents of essential oils, and from those terpenes larger molecules such as steroids. The biochemical clues to this activity are the triterpenes found in the cell walls of the first life forms, prokaryotic cells. Prokaryotes, still encountered today, comprise many species of bacteria, among them friendly bacteria such as the lactobacilli as well as pathogens such as mycobacterium tuberculosis. Prokaryotes are a life form with the simplest schematic blueprint. The prokaryotic cell does not have separations into distinct compartments, instead all biochemical processes happen in one assembly hall. Prokaryotic cells reproduce only asexually, by reduplication. In eukaryotic cells, which appeared at the earliest 1.4 billion years ago, we encounter a more complex organization. Eukaryotic mitochondria and chloroplasts are symbiotically integrated into the biochemical factory we call the cell, forming distinct departments with a distinct head office, the nucleus. These units produce specific substances and are separated from each other by membranes. Eukaryotes developed great diversity and are found in the animal, fungi, and plant kingdoms.

But let us return to the very beginning of life, the simplest organisms: the prokaryotes. The triterpene molecules found in

Table 3.1: Basil species, properties, and indications

Variety	**Active Molecules**	**Properties**	**Indications**
Ocimum basilicum var. *basilicum* (exotic type)	methyl chavicol, linalool, eugenol	antispasmodic, active on sympathicus, antiinflammative, antiviral	gastritis, pancreatic insufficiency, viral hepatitis A & B, travel sickness, prostatitis, urinary tract infections
Ocimum basilicum var. *European* (linalool type)	cis-3-hexenol, linalool, fenchol, eugenol, methyl chavicol, 1.8-cineole	tonifying, carminative, hepatostimulant, neurotonic	coronary weakness, nervous depression, liver, gall insufficiency
Ocimum basilicum var. *grand vert*	methyl chavicol, methyl eugenol, ß-caryophyllene	strongly antispasmodic	colitis, spasmophilia
Ocimum basilicum var. *minimum*	methyl chavicol, methyl eugenol, ß-caryophyllene, neral, alpha & beta pinenes, citronellal, geranial	antispasmodic, antiinfectious	spasmodic colitis

Table 3.1, continued

Variety	Active Molecules	Properties	Indications
Ocimum gratissimum (eugenol type)	cis- & trans-ß-ocimenes, ß-caryophyllene, alpha & beta santalene, eugenol, methyl chavicol	antiinfectious, bactericidal, viricidal, parasiticidal, neurotonic, hormone-like	enterocolitis, intestinal parasitosis, hepatopancreatic insufficiency, prostata congetion, arthrosis
Ocimum gratissimum (thymol type)	paracymene, alpha thujene, myrcene	general stimulant, strongly antiinfectious	cystitis, bronchitis, enterocolitis

prokaryotic outer cell walls have a tetracyclic structure that imparts rigidity and acts as a mechanical-stabilizing or wall-forming agent. Triterpenes are molecules built along the same biochemical assembly line as the terpenes, only they are three times as large, containing not ten but thirty carbon atoms. As life evolved, different marine algae developed that again contained compounds made by the identical biosynthetic pathway.

But life as we know it could not have happened with aromatic and steroid molecules alone. Proteins, sugars, and fats are all present in simple cells today as they were four billion years ago.

Algae, mosses, and mushrooms

We do not know, in terms of the earth's history, exactly when fungi appeared, but many species contain terpene compounds and essential oils. Mosses and lichens are known to have existed since the upper Devonian period, approximately 350 million years ago, although some scientists speculate that they might be older. In

Figure 3.1:
Phylogenic development of plants: Selected species and representative molecules of their secondary metabolism

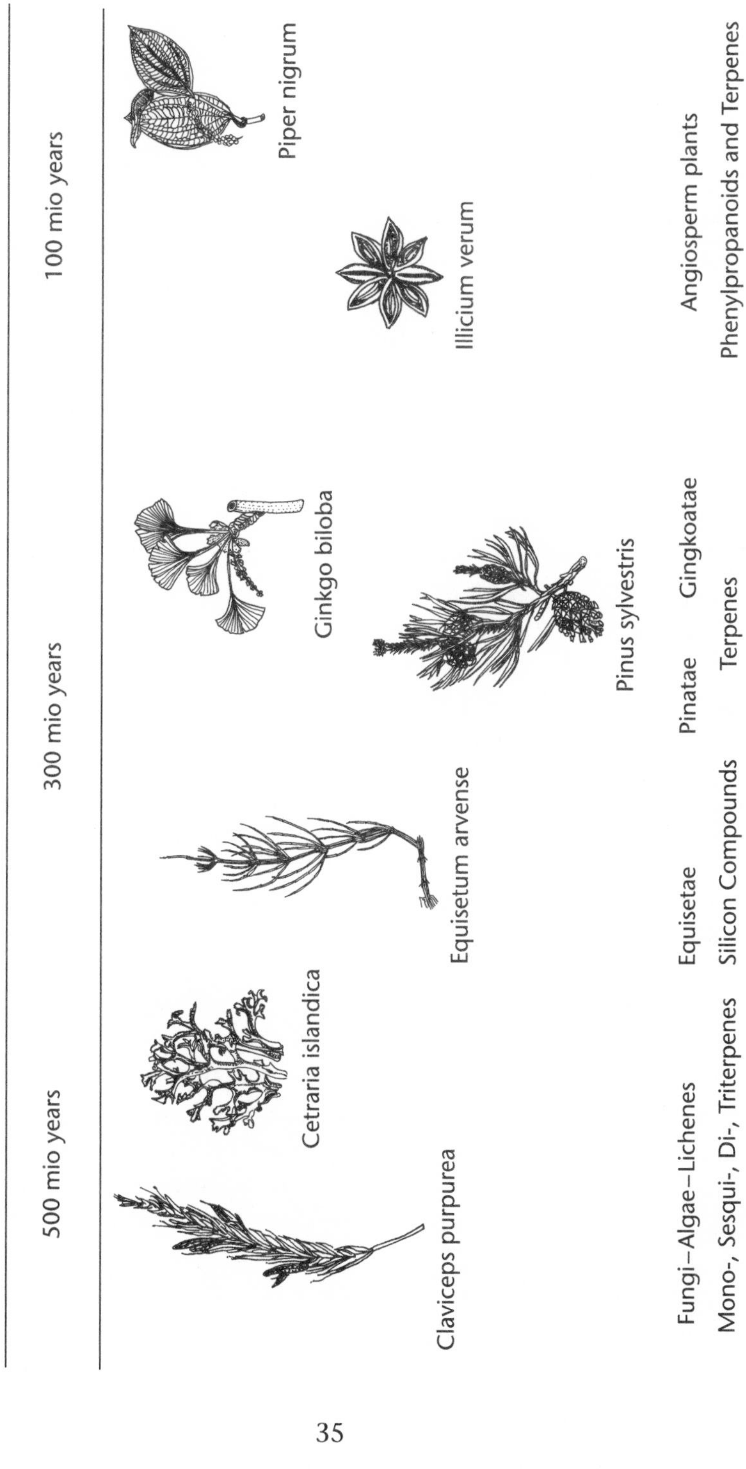

500 mio years		300 mio years		100 mio years
Claviceps purpurea	Cetraria islandica	Equisetum arvense	Pinus sylvestris, Ginkgo biloba	Illicium verum, Piper nigrum
Fungi–Algae–Lichenes		Equisetae	Pinatae, Gingkoatae	Angiosperm plants
Mono-, Sesqui-, Di-, Triterpenes		Silicon Compounds	Terpenes	Phenylpropanoids and Terpenes

their biochemistry, mosses and lichens bear some resemblance to ferns and seeded plants, which appeared when life migrated out of the water, but the differences lie in their membranous substances.

Mosses contain phenolic compounds such as cinnamic acid, which are degradation products of lignin (wood). They also have distinct "containers," which typically store a mixture of essential oil and resinoid substances. The volatile odorants found in mosses are principally monoterpenes, many of which are found in plants that evolved later. Among them are the hydrocarbons limonene and pinene, the monoterpene alcohols geraniol and borneol, aldehydic and ketonic components, and esters such as linalyl and bornyl acetates. A wide range of sesquiterpene structures is also found among these odorants. The characteristic blue coloring of oil containers in *Calypogeia trichomanis* moss is caused by azulene sesquiterpenes. Many of the sesquiterpenes found in mosses are enantiomers of the identical compounds that we find in plants that evolved later. To round out the range of aromatic substances in mosses, we find sesquiterpene lactones and a fair number of diterpenes—some known from other plants and some specific to mosses. Triterpenes are rare, but sterols, especially stigmasterol and sitosterol, are encountered.

Land plants

Approximately 400 million years ago, the first land plants (*Psylophytatae*, or ferns) appeared. These so-called primitive life forms no longer exist, but fifty million years later, *Lycopodiatae* (it is odd that a plant as ancient as *Lycopodium europeum* contains molecules effective against a disease as brand-new, on an evolutionary scale, as hyperthyroidism), *Equisetae* (horsetail) and *Filicatae* (ferns) started populating the earth and some representatives of these phyla of plants still thrive. By analyzing the compounds found in ferns, we can conclude that at this evolutionary stage of plants, the terpene assembly line inside the cell remained intact. Some sesquiterpenes—pterosines—found in ferns have been studied more intensely for their toxic and carcinogenic effects.

Table 3.2: The most important types of aromatic molecules encountered in essential oil bearing plants and their most important properties for aromatherapy

Molecules	**Properties**	**Essential Oils**
Terpenes	stimulant, antiviral, potentially irritant	most citrus and needle oils
Alcohols	tonifying, energizing, antibactrial, antiviral, antifungal, germicidal	*Eucalyptus radiata, Ravensara,* niaouli marjoram, *Rosemary* officinalis, peppermint, geranium, cypress
Phenols	bactericidal, strongly stimulant, potentially irritant	thyme, oregano, savory
Aldehydes	sedative, antiviral, antiinflammtive	*Lemon verbena,* melissa, *Litsea cubeba, Eucalyptus citriodora*
Esters	active on the central nervous system	lavender, clary sage, mandarin, petitgrain, Roman chamomile
Ketones	mucolytic, cell regenerative, potentially neurotoxic	*Rosemary verbenone,* sage, *Thuja, Hyssop* officinalis, Everlast
Oxides	expectorant	*Eucalyptus globulus,* bay laurel, *Hyssop decumbens, Rosemary cineol*
Sesquiterpenes	antiinflammative, antiallergic	German chamomile, Moroccan chamomile
Sesquiterpene alcohols	Liver and glandular stimulant	frankincense, myrrh, patchouli
Sesquiterpene lactones	mucolytic	Inula graveolens

Table 3.2, continued

Molecules	Properties	Essential Oils
Phenyl propanes (hot)	immune stimulant, antibacterial, potentially irritant	clove, cinnamon, oregano, savory
Phenyl propanes (soft)	antispasmodic, balances the central nervous system	anis, basil, tarragon

Needle trees

Three hundred million years ago, essential oils as we know them today were the ubiquitous secondary substances in the coniferous needle trees. At this stage of development, it proved successful for these plants to produce essential oils made predominantly of monoterpenes. Because of the needle trees, we know that limonene, pinene, borneol, carvacrol, and thymol, among others, have figured prominently in the chemistry of life on this planet. Some trees that were prolific in this period are: *Ginkgo biloba* and the *Coniferae, Picea abies, Abies alba, Pseudotsuga menziesii* (North American Douglas fir), *Pinus sylvestris, Pinus pumilio, Sequoia sempervirens, Thuja occidentalis, Juniperus* ssp., and *Cupressus sempervirens*. Relatively unique among these ancient trees, the *Cupressus* species accumulate more essential oil and less balsamic or resinous aromatic substances than other needle trees. The oils of *Cupressaceae* needles contain mono, sesqui, and diterpenes, and the wood oil contains thymol and carvacrol. With the current trend toward esotericism in aromatherapy, it is surprising that there is not yet a range of prehistoric aromatics on the market.

The breakthrough of the herbaceous and the leafy green plants

On the scale of botanical evolution, angiosperms—plants with hulled or covered seeds—are relatively modern. One hundred million years ago these plants started to develop a broad new range of chemical tricks and strategies, and survived to become the most successful form of plants thus far. This was accomplished with the help of a vastly increased variety of products that rolled off the existing biochemical assembly line of terpenes and phenylpropanoids. At the beginning of this development, the less highly organized angiosperms, plants of slightly older development, contained essential oils predominantly made up of products from the shikimic acid pathway (phenylpropanoids). The "shikimic acid pathway" is a biochemical term summarizing a different synthetic pathway line within the plant cell, in which an amino acid, normally intended for the manufacture of proteins, is sidetracked and used as starting material for the manufacture of essential oil components. This amino acid, phenylalanine, is converted into cinnamic acid and from there to phenylpropanoid molecules. Representative plants are star anise, ylang ylang, cinnamon, and nutmeg. In bay laurel we encounter a unique mix of phenylpropanoids and terpenoids.

While different chemical compositions improved the odds for survival, plants were not limited to one set of components per species, such as one set of components for lavender and another set for rosemary. To the contrary, as the example of basil demonstrates, closely related or different populations of identical species answered varying challenges (altitude, climate, soil, herbivores) with different chemical makeups. An early example among the angiosperms is the fact that different populations of *Cinnamomum camphora* established the rather sophisticated principle of chemical races, or in aromatherapy parlance, "chemotypes."[2] Depending on its origin, this plant produces essential oils commercially known as either camphor, ravensara, or ho oil.[11] The chemical differences between the different kin are greater than what might result from climatic or geographic variation alone; they have become genetically fixed.

The botanical origins of medicine

As angiosperms developed even higher degrees of organization, their essential oil composition changed toward a predominance of terpenoid components—which make up approximately 80 percent of all essential oil matter today—and the array of their chemical devices became ever more sophisticated. Throughout one hundred million years of angiosperm evolution, most compounds medicinally important today (including benzylisochinoline and indole alkaloids, lignanes, tannins, irioids, saponines, and so on) were

Table 3.3: Chemotypes of Cinnamomum camphora

Chemical Race	Vernacular Name
Safrole	Camphor
Camphor	Cinnamonum camphor
Cineole	Ravensara aromatica
Linalole	Ho

generated. These substances had already been part of the biology of the planet for hundreds of millions of years when, approximately five million years ago, the first hominids began to roam the earth. Finally, *Homo sapiens,* with a developed frontal cortex, came approximately 120 thousand years ago.[3] Humans thus developed on a cellular basis that had been explored by plants and animals for *much* longer than human existence, which is the most compelling reason to view these chemicals as part and parcel of our own biological makeup.

Conservation

In aromatherapy and medicine, the substances we are mainly concerned with are secondary products of plant organisms. Primary substances are those which are directly involved in the plant's existence and metabolism. Examples of primary substances are: DNA storing genetic information, chlorophyll transforming light energy into chemical energy, and lignins (in wood) providing structure. Secondary substances are made by plants to interact with their environment, to attract pollinators, to repel herbivores, to improve the odds in the competition with other life forms for resources, or for just plain survival. These latter substances were crucial to the drama of life as it played out over the course of evolution. Species came and disappeared, but the cellular principles of chemical manufacturing enjoyed enormous priority in conservation. Substances like alpha pinene or steroids remained the same. The same degree of conservation is encountered in other areas of cellular biology. An astounding example is the human opiate receptor. Given mankind's long history of drug and especially opiate use, it is reasonable to speculate that there is a receptor in our cellular makeup that reacts to opiate substances mediating the known effects of opiate drugs. That the same opiate receptor also exists in insects and invertebrate is more surprising and shows that there are constants in cellular existence that were effectively preserved throughout evolution.

Similarly, the gonadotropic hormone LHRH, one of a number of hormones that regulate sexual desire and reproduction, is found in the simplest and in the most complex organisms, a clear indication that reproductive behavior and the corresponding emotions are being conserved extremely rigidly.[4] The same is probably true for steroids that fulfill many different roles in the cybernetics of organisms and are present in some of the most ancient life forms. These chemical and biological systems have the ability to adapt to rapid changes; they were thrown off course by neither the disappearance of dinosaurs nor by the ice ages.

Evolutionary substances versus twentieth-century pharmacology

Modern science's attempts to improve upon nature should be

viewed against the backdrop of systems that have preserved life for billions of years. There are some who feel that most science and technology no longer improves anything. As far as chemistry and medicine are concerned, there are very few inventions as useful as some of the early ones, such as glass-making.

We read almost daily how virtually every scientific or technological advance backfires in major ways: chlorofluorocarbons deplete the ozone layer, DDT accumulates in the food chain, chemically altered foods are found to be carcinogenic, radioactive and worldwide industrial chemical pollution are rampant, "electrosmog" and mercury fillings cause leukemia, food-processing practices lead to increasing rates of cancer, and almost every single medicine that promises relief actually offers dependence and horrific side effects.

Coming to grips with the fallout from the technological age is hotly discussed in the literature on current affairs. The fact that human and botanical biosystems have remained in place *thus far* leads to the assumption that continued reliance on them might prove more successful than current scientific mythology is willing to admit. Overconfidence in scientific human achievement leads to chemical and biological destruction. But instead of waking up, *"Homo scientificus"* becomes more and more shortsighted and presumptuous with the acceleration of every facet of life.

This shortsightedness is expressed by our very limited view of history, which commonly reflects on only the last two thousand years. Thousands of years of high civilizations like the Egyptian or Chinese cultures are virtually ignored. The epidemic of this type of preposterousness is encountered in the writings of Erich von Dänecken, who contends that the pyramids simply could not have been built by the Egyptians, that they had to have assistance from outer space. What von Dänecken forgets is how much we have been brainwashed on the topic of space travel and, more importantly, that the Egyptian culture was a civilization at its peak, with thousands of years of development behind it. A more sensible and less self-absorbed outlook may be seen in a dialogue from Plato's *Critias* in which an Egyptian sage tells a new immigrant to the

Greek isles that since they had just recently arrived, the Greeks were, naturally, devoid of culture. The sage was able to recall historical events of the Egyptian civilization that reached almost as far back as the last ice age.

Throughout most previous cultures, plant aromatics were intimately involved in defining human identity and individuality, influencing our mating behavior as well as our whole emotional being. At the dawn of recorded history, aromatic substances already were the substances of choice for ritual and magic. Medicinal and religious applications were identical and cultures knew how to use and respect them. Difficult as it may be for Western man (and perhaps less so for Western women) to return to a belief system where the unified use of aromatic plants is the norm, it is high hubris and self-deception to believe that plants stopped working right around the time of World War II just because antibiotics and cortisone became available on an industrial scale.

The biosynthetic blueprint, manifested in the human body with monoterpenes, essential oils, geranyl pyrophosphates, and farnesyl pyrophosphates, existed long before there were humans. This blueprint existed before the great success of the angiosperms and even before the essential oil-producing *Coniferae* made their big splash. It is an archaic chemical pathway that has, like the other biochemical pathways of life, existed since the dawn of life on planet earth.

Aromatic chemical communication systems

A fascinating expression of this planetary chemical system are the biological communication systems that are based on these substances. Coevolution of plants and herbivores is at the origin of these chemical communication systems. For instance, plant constituents, which convey the smell of food, will attract both genders and thereby guide potential sexual partners to the feeding place where the attractant is found. Animals, over time, have learned to mimic such signals by storing and releasing the same or similar compounds, attracting potential mates or deterring rivals. Animals employ metabolites of food (or appropriate imitations) to send chemical messages because they are easily decoded by the receiver. Indeed, striking similarities are found between volatiles from animals and plants.

Terpenes: chemical signals in the air

Almost all types of chemical signals, from sex pheromones to highly potent defense substances, are found among molecules originating from the terpenoid biosynthetic pathway. These molecules are also called mevalogenins because their biosynthesis starts from a common precursor: mevalonic acid.[5]

Monoterpenes are highly important in the communication systems of different insect species. Plant substances participate in host selection in intricate ways. The pine beauty moth distinguishes between different ratios of aromatic compounds (alpha-pinene and beta-pinene) in selecting its oviposition site. In a variation on the theme, alpha-pinene and beta-pinene are part of the alarm pheromones of certain aphid species. In insect societies these compounds are often secreted to achieve group goals: the soldiers of some termite species secrete a sequence of monoterpene hydrocarbons, including limonene, from their frontal glands. Workers of some ant species secrete the same components from their poison glands. Generally, bees, ants, and particularly termites use monoterpene hydrocarbons for defense, reflecting the history they share with needle trees. Monoterpenes containing oxygen, and especially monoterpene esters, are more fruity and floral in aroma and are abundant in bees in part because of their close contact with flowers. Typical flower volatiles such as nerol, geraniol, citral, citronellol, and linalool are widespread in the insect world and are part of basic survival mechanisms: citronellol is a male sex attractant of the two-spotted spider mite; stingless bees secrete large amounts of citral during their raids to disorientate prey bee species while plundering their nests; Centris bees deposit a mixture of monoterpenes on grass stems to mark territories; and nerolic and geranic acids, combined with nerol and citral, have been identified in a pheromone that plays a role in worker-bee attraction, nest finding, foraging, and marking of food sources. For these insects, essential-oil components are fundamental molecules of communication.

Another example is the bark beetle. The males release compounds attracting both sexes of the species in order to induce a mass attack on a selected tree and overcome the tree's resistance by mass colonization. Generally, insects that attack conifers must overcome the physical and chemical defenses of the tree during colonization. Exuding sticky and toxic oleoresins is the tree's most effective means of warding off bark beetle invasion. However, the bark beetles successfully adapted their strategies: they utilize the

Figure 3.2: Dominant terpenes in needle trees

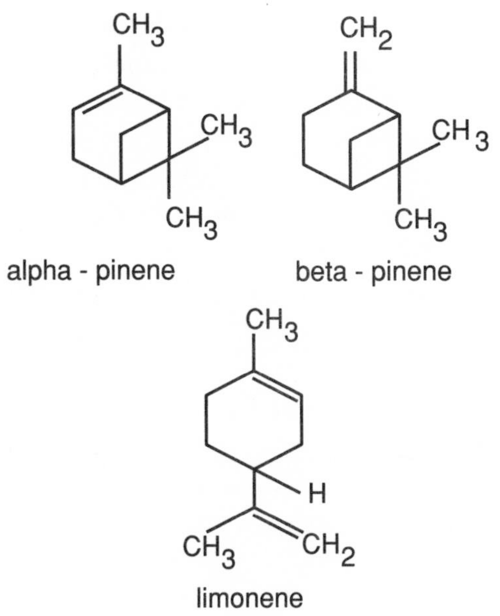

CH_3 CH_3 CH_3

alpha - pinene

CH_2 CH_3 CH_3

beta - pinene

CH_3 H CH_3 CH_2

limonene

monoterpenes found in resinous compounds of the host trees to summon their own forces.

The compound secreted by the male bark beetle to attract both species is secreted by hornets to induce alarm among workers. This compound was also found among the volatiles of citrus fruits and hops and has a strong narcotic effect on mice. A sesquiterpene found in the essential oil of certain tropical plants, where it acts as a toxic deterrent to leaf-cutting ants, is also a major component of the secretion of the swallowtail moth larvae. Modified rose oxide is a defense compound secreted by the common grasshopper.

These examples illustrate that nature uses the same substances over and over. They are part of the chemistry of living cells. Natural processes prefer to modify existing concepts or mix existing compounds in specific ratios. That citronellol, nerol, and linalool have been successfully employed for the most diverse needs of living organisms is a clear indication of their effectiveness. The conventional scientific view implies that essential-oil compounds are no different from those synthesized in the lab. The deep involvement of these substances in cellular processes disproves this outright. Essential-oil compounds are among the molecules of life itself. They are produced by living organisms and remain present in living organisms, even acting in the interest of the organism's survival. To approach these botanical components as mere random chemicals with little or no effect is one of the more successful pieces of propaganda that corporate-funded science has generated. If any amount of intensified research was performed to demonstrate the effectiveness of these natural molecules, perhaps this picture would change drastically.

This can be concluded from the results of the little research that has been performed. An example is the data on cinnamic aldehyde, which is effective against most pathogenic intestinal bacteria but does not inhibit or attack streptococcus faecalis, a bacterium often counted among the beneficial or harmless passenger organisms in the intestines.[6] That cinnamic aldehyde and other phenylpropanoids can distinguish between pathogenic and friendly bacteria is a clear example how these molecules of life act much more cooperatively than do random lab substances. That is why they persisted through evolution—without specific and finely tailored benefits, they would have disappeared.

Lipophilic messengers

Candace Pert's *The Molecules of Emotion* makes clear how much aromatherapy stands to gain from the evolving field of psycho-neuro immunology. The book explains the astounding shifts that have occurred in the world of science with the discovery of receptors and neurotransmitters, and reveals the all-encompassing ways that these systems govern the action of practically every organ in the body. In Pert's words, "...it does not matter if you were a lab rat, a first lady or a dope addict, everyone has the exact same mechanism in the brain for creating bliss and expanded consciousness."

As receptor research progresses, the conservation of the chemistry of transmitter or hormonal molecules becomes increasingly acknowledged by science. This is still not the case for aromatic substances. For an improved understanding of their mechanisms of action we must, in the absence of deftly funded mainstream research, let our fantasies wander. At the beginning of evolution, when life developed in water, molecules that transmitted information and emotion (the neurotransmitters), had to be viable in water. This means that these molecules had to be highly polar to be compatible with or even soluble in water. The peptide neurotransmitters, made up of small numbers of highly polar amino acids, fulfilled that condition. But as land plants established themselves, air became available as a medium for transmission of information. This was a time when small, lipophilic, volatile molecules, aromatherapy's essential oils, had their day in evolution. They could travel through air and interact with organisms and possibly their receptors at great distances.

The structure of the simple phenylpropanoid molecules found in essential oils is similar to some known transmitters. These phenylpropanoids may not be tailored exactly to these receptors, but they could be "loose fits." If the phenylpropanoids do not attach very strongly to receptors, they might bind reversibly, which means that they keep bouncing on and off the receptor. This hypothesis would explain why aromatherapy treatments are often so effective for individuals who use little or no allopathic drugs. If harder-hitting allopathic substances are present, binding to receptors more strongly or irreversibly, they may effectively block the phenylpropanoids. Because another substance is blocking access, aromatics may not have a chance to interact with the receptor and initiate their normal biological effects. Aromatic molecules can be seen as the lipophilic counterpart to the polar peptide transmitters, the "molecules of emotion." Discoveries about the interaction between terpenes, sesquiterpenes, and receptors support this assumption and are discussed in Chapter 6.

"If as a chemist, I see a flower, I know all that is involved in synthesizing a flower's elements. And I know that even the fact that it exists is not something that is natural. It is a miracle."
—Albert Hofmann

FOUR

The Vitalist/Physicalist Debate

Hard sciences in aroma research

When scientific publications or databases are searched for research on aromatherapy, very little, if anything, is found. What is found pertains to a rather narrow definition of aromatherapy given by G. Buchbauer: "...therapeutic uses of fragrances or at least mere volatiles to cure and to mitigate or to prevent diseases, infections and indispositions only by means of inhalation."[1] Aromatherapy is merely the effect of perceiving a fragrance? This definition is weak because it produces contradictions immediately. Even though inhalation is mentioned in the definition, the physical consequence of inhalation, absorption, and the resulting effects are not part of this interpretation of aromatherapy. This highly idiosyncratic view of aromatherapy never took hold. Confining aromatherapy to the physical effects of perceiving aroma is entirely out of touch with the developments aromatherapy has taken in the real world. Throughout its history, aromatherapy has been and still is the therapeutic utilization of essential oils. Buchbauer's semantic trickery is flattened by the term that defines his field of expertise: "organic" chemistry. The term remains in place despite the fact that the field has grown beyond its literal meaning. No one expects organic chemistry to be exclusively the chemistry of substances originating in biological organs, though this is exactly what it originally meant.[2]

To be clear, in this book I will call all forms of therapeutic use of essential oils "aromatherapy" and I shall distinguish aromatherapy from the above-described line of research by occasionally referring to it as "aroma research" and/or "aromachology."

While limiting aromatherapy to fragrance effects poorly defines it, the question of whether smelling fragrances is therapeutic is highly relevant. In his presentation at the 13th International Congress of Flavours, Fragrances and Essential Oils, Buchbauer reviewed the methods with which the physiological effects of the inhalation of odorants are researched. He attempts to draw a clear line of demarcation between his definitions of aromatherapy and aromachology. According to his definition, "aromatherapy" (which should be referred to as "aroma research" or "fragrance therapy") is where the perception of an aroma creates a physiological and/or pharmacological effect, whereas "aromachology" studies the relationship of psychology and odors.

Measuring the physiological effects of fragrance perception

Buchbauer's group showed that lavender oil, its main constituents linalool and linalyl acetate, neroli oil, citronellal (a constituent of citronella oil), alpha terpineol, benzaldehyde, and east Indian sandalwood oil all decreased the motility of mice, even when they were agitated by caffeine.[3] Methods to quantify the effects of odorants on physiological parameters include the measurement of skin potential levels (SPL), which are related to mental activity and correspond with the arousal level of a test person.[4] Measuring SPLs via contingent negative variation (CNV), S. Torii found that chamomile sedated and jasmine stimulated his subjects. Skin potential levels changed parallel to the activity of the sympathetic nervous system. This indicates that pleasant as well as unpleasant odors raise arousal levels and that especially unpleasant odors cause large fluctuations in SPLs.

CNV is the slow upward shift in brain waves that is recorded by an electroencephalogram (EEG) and occurs when test persons are tense or in anticipation of something. Torii was the first to use this method to investigate the physiological effects of odorants on humans. He showed that jasmine oil caused an increase in CNV similar to that caused by caffeine, while lavender oil decreased CNV like a tranquilizer. What this research really says is that essential oils produce changes when CNV is measured. To say that the effects of oils are similar to caffeine or tranquilizers simply because those also have an effect on CNV measurements would be somewhat of a stretch.

In a later work by Kubota et al., these results were basically confirmed. However, new twists were added to the investigations. They measured the CNV of whole essential oils, but continued their research by fractionating the essential oils into three parts: a light boiling fraction composed mainly of volatile monoterpene hydrocarbons, and two fractions of higher boiling components that would most likely represent sesquiterpene components. They found that sometimes one component of an oil was stimulating while another component of the same oil was sedating. In conventional parlance, these seemingly contradictory observations amount to *no* effect. In the holistic viewpoint, essential oils combine different effects into one synergy. This research points to the problems the reductionist method has with the complex effects of fragrances on a human being. The results of the studies, that jasmine stimulates and chamomile sedates, are not new. It is considered an "achievement" that a method was found that could bestow some form of scientific proof on something that was long known traditionally and almost as a matter of common sense!

Another method employed to observe the physiological effects of odorants is termed "plethysmography." This method allows the observation of changes in the peripheral bloodstream caused by the sympathetic component of the autonomic nervous system. Plethysmography can show modulating effects of odorants on the symptoms of stress, such as the constriction of the peripheral capillaries, which increases blood pressure. With this method it was possible to demonstrate that peppermint can initiate a neurophysiological illusioning of stress (constriction) and that jasmine produces relaxation (dilation).[7] Physiological effects of odorants on heart rate can also be observed when distinct differences between stimulating and sedating odorants exist.

No simple or clear picture emerges when all these different experiments are compared. The finding that jasmine is stimulating *and* relieves induced stress points to the rather crude nature of the employed methods. Buchbauer concludes simply that a variety of different methods have been employed in aromatherapy research to demonstrate the healing or physiological effects of essential oils.

"Aromachology is a young discipline. The picture...is complex, confusing and in part contradictory." This quote is, for effect, taken out of context from an excellent review by Dr. J. S. Jellinek. In this review, Jellinek surveys the existing literature on aromachology and also clarifies some important issues about aromatherapy.[8]

The disciplines of aromatherapy and aromachology overlap in many areas and it is often difficult to decide where one starts and the other ends. Reviewing the historical development helps to clarify the situation. Aromatherapy, the healing discipline that uses essential oils in the tradition of Gattefossé, Valnet, and Tisserand, existed first. Then, suddenly, exciting new smell and fragrance research received increased attention. "Olfaction" became fashionable and aromatherapy conferences featured olfaction and fragrance research as much as classic aromatherapy. One reason for this crossover was that the usually veritable academic credentials of the fragrance researchers lent weight to the conference lineup. But CNV research that showed increased alertness as a result of lemon oil leaves many aromatherapists strangely untouched. Jellinek's review recognizes the need for and proposes the necessary distinction between aromatherapy and aromachology.

A significant difference between aromachology and aromatherapy is their respective position toward special virtues of *natural* odorants. Jellinek continues: "The basic distinction is made right along the substances which both disciplines are concerned with. Classical aromatherapy ascribes special virtues to natural essential oils and works predominantly with these oils." He goes on to say that "there is no evidence of any general or fundamental difference between the different categories of stimuli with respect to their aromachology effects." Jellinek clearly does not say that there aren't *any* different effects, he candidly states that there aren't any with respect to aromachology. This again follows directly from the scientific definition of aromachology, in which the main thrust is to measure a response—any response—and synthetics can create responses just as well as natural substances. The differences lie in the quality of the response: vitalists believe that the response to natural materials is generally benign or positive and that synthetics have a much higher likelihood of causing adverse effects. Physicalists believe that no such assumptions can be made on the basis of the natural or synthetic nature of a substance.

Essential oils were used at least since the Renaissance for emotional uplifting, for improving mental activity, and for strengthening memory. The question raised by much of the aromachology research is: Does aromachology confirm or disprove historical claims of aromatherapy in this area? In Jellinek's words: "A dispassionate look at the evidence leads to the conclusion that aromatherapy's attribution of facts have been verified in several instances, but to a rather restricted degree." But he also considers the aromatherapy standpoint: "There is, however, an alternative way to look at the situation. The removal of interfering variables, a necessity in the contemporary scientific tradition in which aromachology is embedded, is foreign to the tradition of aromatherapy."

Holism sells

By turning aroma*therapy* into aroma*chology*, introducing the scientific viewpoint and requiring proof the reductionist way, a familiar trend is set in motion. Things or procedures like aromatherapy, which start as cottage industry and serve human needs, begin to grow economically. Increased acceptance and legitimacy tend to follow whenever larger corporations become involved in aromatherapy. What is lost in the excitement is that the priorities shift. Aromatherapy from then on will serve the needs of the corporation first and human needs second. The original intent, to benefit people, becomes a hollow front; the real driving force is the expectation of exploiting this budding therapy. Jellinek says as much:

> The idea to employ environmental fragrances to enhance specific emotional states and predispositions is by no means new. The use of scent in temples and at religious ceremonies, at feasts and celebrations, and for the promotion of love goes back as far as recorded history. What is new are the specific applications being suggested today: They reflect the needs and priorities of our times. New and again typical of our age is also the scientific spirit of controlled experimentation and statistical analysis which aromachology brings to bear upon this field. Aromachology [science] is used to establish the justification of claims, aromatherapy [holistic reasoning] is used to market a product's purpose to the consumer. One may take exception to this intertwining of fundamentally different perspectives, but it is standard practice in many fields including, for example, medicine. It is, in fact, the best way we have today of developing and marketing products that are both effective and successful.

In our current economic system this should not be surprising. One would almost expect growth-oriented fragrance companies to try and conquer as much as possible of an evolving market. After all, conventional medicine limits access to the health-care market to deep corporate pockets by implementing expensive, reductionist hurdles known as the drug approval processes. A similar development in the aroma arena, where smells would be proven effective by reductionist means and then sold under the guise of clever, wholesome-sounding marketing may be around the corner. Consumers need to understand that industry-sponsored aromachology research really is meant to benefit business first and is not an exercise in holistic healing, nor does it advance humanity. This is ironic, because the broadening interest in olfaction and fragrance was originally sparked by the resurgence of aromatherapy.

The esoteric approach

> "I was aware of my physical body responding in such a way to the smelling of Khella oil that I had never experienced. "Clearing" is the only way I describe a very powerful, quick and thorough sensation, right through my physical body and on into my energetic fields, to experience 'white out' in my aura."[9]

First-hand accounts like this one from a popular aromatherapy quarterly represent the other extreme in the assessment of fragrance effects. For those who grew up with an unchallenged belief in the scientific manner of explaining the world, this might be too much to stomach. But it is experiences like this that stimulate exploration of the effects of essential oils. In the absence of big science, experience is a big part of contemporary aromatherapy reality. Still, uneasiness remains. Later in the same article, the reason becomes obvious. It is not the lack of scientific demeanor but the heightened need for medical help that lends itself to this kind of language. The article, entitled "A Case for Khella," cites several cases. The one quoted here is Case B, Liver Cancer:

> Client had liver cancer and was to receive chemotherapy. However, her immunology count was very low, only 0.4%, so treatment was canceled. Her aromatherapist was "inspired" to make up a blend of khella oil in a base of Manuka. The client sniffed the bottle only when moved to do so. Four days later, her immunology count was back up to 5, so the chemotherapy could take place. The client continued to sniff the blend when she felt the need, which lessened progressively.

Coumarins are among the more pharmacologically active components found in essential oils. Often they are strongly polar and/or their molecular weights are such that they are only encountered in low concentrations. Chemically speaking, they are benzo alpha pyrones, or compounds that are derived from these. The word "coumarin" originates from the coumarouna tree from Guyana, South America, Dipteryx odorata. Out of its seeds, tonka beans, the first nonsubstituted benzo alpha pyrone was isolated in crystallized form. It is distinguished from nonsubstituted coumarins, which are colorless crystalline compounds with a characteristic fragrance. This compound is encountered widely among different angiosperms. Often coumarins are present in the plant bound to sugar molecules. Only when the plant is cut and dried does the coumarin break away from this larger molecule and become present in the plant as such. This is observed when grass is cut and creates the distinct fragrance of fresh-mown hay.

Coumarins are typical secondary products of plant metabolism that, in low concentrations, have been shown to stimulate the growth of the roots of plants. Some decades ago, coumarins were used in pharmacology and in the food industry as a flavor and fragrance additive. In animal experiments, however, this practice was found to lead to liver damage and therefore is no longer used today. Various coumarins have antiphlogistic and circulatory stimulant properties. Others are spasmolytic or sedative and can also have bactericidal properties. Some, such as aesculine, are used as venous tonics.

Distinct from the simple coumarins are the furano coumarins. Some representatives are psoralene, bergaptene, xantho toxin, angelicine, and pimpinelline. The furano coumarins are responsible for the photosensitizing effects observed in various oils of the citrus (Rutaceae) and Apiaceae families. Another type of compound is pyranocoumarin. Representatives of this group are compounds found in khella, Ammi visnaga, identified as visnadine, samedine, and dihydrosamedine. Visnadine is useful as a coronary dilator. It is interesting to note that fungi such as aspergillus flavus and others may contain the highly toxic aflatoxin B, which is also a coumarin.[10]

The example above shows the confusion typical of the aromatherapist who wants to treat intuitively but sound scientific. The language gives it away: "Client had liver cancer and was to receive chemotherapy." The omission of an article before "client" gives the report a datalike, scientific, and therefore "true" ring. The arti-

Table 4.1: Active principles, properties, and indications of Ammi visnaga

Active principles	Properties	Indications
Alcohols: linalool, borneol	antispasmodic,	asthma
Esters: bornyl acetate	bronchial, coronary and	liver and kidney colic,
Coumarins	urinary dilator	coronary insufficiency,
Chromones: khelline, visnagine	anticoagulant	athereosclerosis

cle continues, "...her immunology count was very low, only 0.4%..." Point four percent of what? The language is vague but tries to sound scientific.

The urge to simplify and to appeal to instinct is fueled by commercial interests. A rather large target group thirsty for such manufactured lore has gathered under the banner of aromatherapy. This mix of (scientific) truth and fiction (inconclusive conjecture) is an aromatherapist's schizophrenia. Reversing the predicament of big business, the young field of aromatherapy wants to invoke science to appear official and ultimately to sell.

The text continues: in precisely four days, the client's "immunology count," purportedly as a result of sniffing khella oil, "...was back up to 5, so the chemotherapy could take place."

Ultimately it is always each individual's choice how to manage relentless, life-threatening, and challenging circumstances such as cancer. It is certainly everyone's prerogative to resort to conventional, allopathic medical offerings when reason, hope, or fear dictate. But to see a return to more allopathic treatment—such as sniffing khella oil only to pave the way for more chemotherapy—celebrated as a success by an advocate of aromatherapy is alarming. Especially in cases like this one, where the allopathic treatment is known to rob patients of their last modicums of dignity, let alone quality of life.

The clash: vitalism versus physicalism

The previous anecdote encompasses the disorientation found in this branch of aromatherapy. It shows that the concepts of vitalism and physicalism are totally muddled. It seems that proponents of this murky thinking may not even be aware of the mutually exclusive nature of vitalist and physicalist philosophy.

Confusion reigns because on one hand there is a strong movement towards the intuitive, which for all practical purposes represents the "New Age" side of aromatherapy, as clearly evidenced by this article. Celebrating intuition is exactly what the readers of such publications expect and it is part of what makes aromatherapy different. This spirited enthusiasm is close to the hearts and minds of those who are passionate about aromatherapy, but it does not bode well for doing business in the health-care arena where the rules are set up by the conventional medical establishment.

Articles in periodicals devoted to aromatherapy show that there is no consensus on the ultimate direction of aromatherapy. A letter to the editor of an Australian aromatherapy journal brings this to the point: "If the aromatherapy profession wants to be respected and acknowledged by the conventional western medicine world, then, whether we like it or not, we have to show substantial and replicable clinical evidence of our claims."[11]

Let us for a moment pretend that this is what we would like to do: show substantial and replicable clinical evidence for the validity of aromatherapy. So far attempts at doing just that have not been very successful. (The reasons will be explored a little further in this chapter.)

In order to get a piece of the health-care action, the "complementary" status has been invented. "Complementary" means that in some circumstances, such as in hospital rooms, nurses are allowed to relieve emotional stress and pep up patients with dosages of essential oils. The establishment considers this quite harmless, but not to be taken seriously. Surveying the predominantly British literature on using aromatherapy for complementary treatments, one recommendation will come up ad infinitum: if a condition gets too serious, one must immediately turn that patient back over to the allopathic system for more pharmaceuticals, which I suspect are at the root of the original problem. The above example of treating a cancer patient shows how a fair amount of cynicism can spring from the complementary approach. Aromatherapy is utilized to improve the condition of patients to the degree that they can undergo more assaults by allopathic medicine.

The British approach

The root of the dichotomy is that there is no true vitalist/physicalist discourse in the influential world of aromatherapy in Great Britain.[14] Considering that many of the aromatherapy organizations and publications in Great Britain regard themselves as opinion-forming entities on a global scale, this situation is disappointing.[12] Given their international influence, it would be even more critical to identify and address the dichotomy: the pursuit of a scientific appearance for a modality with a vitalistic core. Trying to substantiate the validity of aromatherapy by integrating often rather indiscriminate arrays of scientific factoids is a common style in contemporary aromatherapy writing. Such writers draw on the well-intentioned premise that, through scientific proof, aromatherapy will gain mainstream acceptance ("whether we like it or not we have to show substantial and replicable clinical evidence"). This hope will ultimately be disappointed because it is not scientific proof but economic realities that determine acceptance or nonacceptance. (More on this in Chapter 5.)

Aromatherapy's ambivalent relation to science

What is needed is a theoretical framework that provides a platform from which aromatherapy can develop in a self-confident manner without constantly worrying whether outside authorities approve or not. The first element of such a platform is a clarification of the relationship aromatherapy has with science.

Scientific exploration of essential-oil constituents and their effects is a valuable tool. Its pursuit can be an important part of aromatherapy, contributing to the knowledge about the pharmacology of oils and their quasi-medicinal applications. Scientific exploration will not be able to explain the *living* nature of essential oils from plants, as by its own admission the scientific paradigm operates from an assumption that the universe is "dead matter in space."[13] The hegemony of the scientific paradigm is built on the latter premise and therefore squarely denies that there is anything special in an oil except its being composed of random chemicals.

This paradoxical situation characterizes so much of what goes on in today's world in general, in medicine, and in dealing with alternative modalities. The concepts of reductionist experimentation have taken on such dominance that only those realities open to this mode of experimentation are considered real. Phenomena too complex for this method are arrogantly declared irrelevant.

Inherent problems with the study of fragrance

The reductionist method simply is not very useful to make relevant statements about such complex areas as fragrance and identity. But the appeal and the reality of aromatherapy thrive on the realization that there are realities different from those conveniently described by science. These realties form the second and third element of an independent aromatherapy. These include the difficulty to quantify aspects of individuality and odor, and the strengthened fabric of life that results from strengthened individuality. In a scientifically correct aromachology experiment, all variables but the one being observed are eliminated. But the hedonic qualities of a flavor or a fragrance exert an influence on the outcome of any experiment. How can liking or disliking a fragrance be eliminated? How unreal is a situation where fragrance has been robbed of its hedonic element, and how relevant can such an experiment be for normal human existence? Obviously the scientific method runs into huge problems when it deals with interconnected phenomena such as fragrance, feeling, and culture. The scientific method will be unable to make meaningful statements in this field as long as it is dependent on measuring the changes of only one variable. In other words, current scientific practice requires that reality is simplified until it becomes measurable. But once that is achieved, is the reality observed the same that was originally intended to be observed? In perfect agreement with Heisenberg's uncertainty principle, results generated by the aromachology observer represent the researchers interference with the object of his observation, not a reality that was present originally.

These issues have not been discussed in aromatherapy publications. New Age-jargon-imbued contributions appear right next to others in which scientifically minded authors pontificate to a public perceived as being uneducated. The hegemony of the mechanistic worldview is never openly stated, but always implied. S. Jellinek raised the issue in his discussion of aromachology. His highly refined way of looking at these complex issues is evident in his choice of words. He seems to be acutely aware that essential oils can do much more than can be scientifically proven. He calls science a contemporary tradition, acknowledging that another age or cultural tradition may choose to look at things differently: "In fact, aromatherapy actively seeks to introduce such variables. Its approach is wholistic." His analysis also acknowledges the accompanying factors (variables) at play during an aromatherapy treatment, including the practitioner's experience and authority, massage or other application method, placebo effects, and many more.

The third element of independent aromatherapy is the recognition that the interaction of aromatherapy with humans cannot be reduced to a single variable experiment. At any given time that an oil interacts with a human being, combined effects of often over a hundred different chemical components initiate different processes all happening simultaneously. Touching soul and spirit, essential oils elicit complex responses from the psychosomatic net-

Table 4.2: The three dimensions of response to fragrance.

Quality of response	Result	Direction
Subjective/Emotional	Hedonic moment	Mood improvement
Behavioral/Mental	Attitude modification	Agression to nonagression
Objective/Physical	Endocrine stimulation	Improved physical health

works of any one person. This quality is unique to the fragrances of nature; it is difficult to conceive that Marcel Proust would have been able to write about today's Day-Glo fragrances the way he wrote about the aromas of his childhood.

The fourth element is found in the new sciences, which understand and allow the existence of psychosomatic networks. These new sciences will provide the aromatherapy treatments and advances of tomorrow by giving insight into the interaction of highly effective sesquiterpene compounds and receptor systems. This new science will ultimately lead to a much improved understanding of why certain aromatic plants were written up in the Sumerian epic of Gilgamesh or in the bible. Being able to rationalize the effects of oils such as myrrh, vetiver, and ginger will create an immediate connection to past cultural uses of these plants. Aromatherapy connects back to the human condition where medicine and religion were not really separable and their unity was more often then not also mediated by aromatics.

I have therefore come to the following conclusions. Aromatherapy is not unscientific, nor does it subscribe to the scientific worldview. For aromatherapy's purposes, science is a tool to advance specialized, factual knowledge about essential oils. But aromatherapy owes its popularity and timeliness to the fact that it has a vitalist core. Almost all of the popular aromatherapy books attribute special powers to true essential oils because, in one way or another, they represent the essence, the soul, or some other height-

Figure 4.2: Five elements of holistic aromatherapy

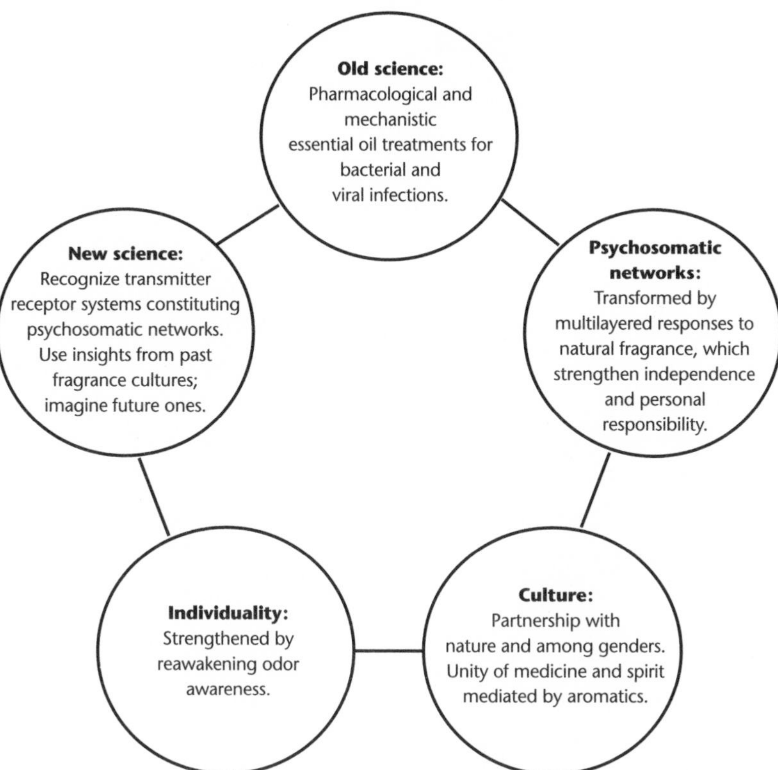

ened principle of the plant. Whatever one's personal convictions, it seems reasonable to state that aromatherapy connects to the phenomena of life much more closely and intimately than does conventional medicine. Essential oils reawaken odor awareness and the connection to individuality, and greater independence improves the ability to take on responsibility for one's own health. Self-confidence and well-being are influenced, providing an improved flow of biological information through the psychosomatic networks of body and mind.

The new sciences, fundamentally different from the old doctrines, understand the reality of psychosomatic networks and they demonstrate the interaction of essential-oil components with these circuits, showing why humanity has integrated these aromatics into its cultures. Aromatherapy is at the center of this new way of thinking. It is the first modality that fully utilizes the advances of science but overcomes its limitations by reintegrating the element of life on every level.

Jellinek, like many seasoned scientists, is fully aware of the limitations of science and the tantamount importance of cultural aspects for all phenomena related to smell. He remarks, with a keen sense for reality and truth, "In view of great inter-individual variance of response, the assumption that a given fragrance works equally for everybody is unwarranted. Until and unless indirect, cognition mediated responses have been excluded, we should, moreover, be wary of applying findings obtained in one country to other countries with different odor cultures."

El sueno de razon produce monstruos."
—Francisco Goya

FIVE
Unhealthy Consequences of the Scientific Revolution

The scientific revolution primer

An inquiry into the origins and progression of the scientific revolution has been done in more or less detail in a number of contemporary writings.[1] This chapter, therefore, shall briefly summarize the phenomenon of science and its consequences. Around the year 1620 René Descartes set out to build the foundations for a new method of understanding with his *Rules for the Direction of the Mind.* His ambition was to describe how the mind worked, and there was no question that for him this task could only be mastered with the tools of mathematics. At the same time, the English philosopher Francis Bacon embarked on an almost identical project. Unlike Descartes, Bacon elected to emphasize the importance of observation and the accumulation of facts. The fusion of these two concepts—Descartes' rationalism and Bacon's empiricism—created a phenomenon now known as science. At the end of the twentieth century, this notion may be genuinely underwhelming, but given that just prior to Descartes' time the church still provided a rigid worldview in which the earth was flat, these were utterly radical approaches. Shortly thereafter, the church-controlled worldview became supplanted by what is now known as the scientific revolution.

As a result, truth changed its quality. Divine right was replaced by what could be measured. Absolute knowledge was only to be found in quantitative data that could be mathematically formulated into laws of physical forces. The first triumph of the new approach were Newton's laws of force, gravitation, and planetary movement. The pioneers of this new paradigm were certain that confused and prejudicial thinking would fade before the scientific clarity and mastery that would provide man with the material and social counterpart to the spiritual redemption offered by God. In Bacon's strong words, nature was now "to be bound into service and made a slave, she [!] would be put upon the rack of scientific investigation and made to reveal her secrets."

Dominator science and sexism

As science celebrated its "triumph" over nature (perceived as female), sexist implications followed directly. Male scientists in a patriarchal world were inebriated by their own grandiosity. The ultimate push of the male scientific mind to subjugate nature cleared all reverence to mother earth and viewed the (usually white) male riding the ultimate road to power straight to the top of the universe. Many authors have recently drawn attention to the blatantly sexist character of the origins of the scientific revolution (Theodore Roszak's *The Voice of the Earth* and *The Memoirs of Elizabeth Frankenstein,* and Charlene Spretnak's *The Resurgence of the Real*). They point to the language of Francis Bacon, which seems equally applicable to his involvement in the courts of inquisition during the witch-hunt trials as to his intellectual arousal regarding putting nature on the rack and torturing her. In Spretnak's words:

> The witch hunts, known today as the Burning Times, spanned the same period as the Reformation and the Scientific Revolution in Britain and on the Continent. As European men asserted their power over the world through the new science and nascent imperialism, they also tightened their control over women. New national laws denied women control of their property and earnings, barred them

> from higher education and professional training, outlawed their efforts to control their own fertility, and placed them under the authority of their husbands. The new modern order was enforced by a system of sexual terrorism, in which hundreds of thousands of women, mostly in the German principalities, were accused of witchcraft, tortured into signing confessions, and then further tortured in a public ritual before being burned at the stake. (Some men were also burned, but in far fewer numbers and for different reasons, usually homosexuality.) Often the women selected for persecution were older women who, while financially dependent, had authority in their communities as healers, midwives, or advisors. Frequently they were outspoken wives, who were considered monstrous shrews or unnatural traitors to their husbands. Certainly the murderous witch-hunts of the sixteenth and seventeenth centuries convinced women to keep a low profile in early modern Europe for many generations thereafter.[2]

Long after the witch-hunts, women are still discriminated against in medicine. While many women have entered medicine, it is still exasperatingly more difficult for women to receive academic honors befitting their scientific or professional achievements. This is especially true in the upper echelons of medicine when the time comes to fill positions in the nation's prestigious medical institutions.[3] The medical profession is still a hostile environment for women doctors and an atmosphere of exclusion persists. Women are forced to redirect their work into more obscure subspecialties and are funneled into clinical practice while men dominate the celebrated and lucrative world of research. Women who attempt both clinical practice and research are usually relegated to second-string clinical research projects and their work is often not formally recognized.

The sexist nature of medicine shows up in what has been termed the "research gap." A thirty-year study of random clinical trials of drug therapy for heart attacks found that fewer than 20 percent of the patients included in the studies were female. In studies of colorectal cancer, which kills more women than all gynecological disorders combined, only 44 percent of the subjects studied were women. Gender bias also persists outside of academia in normal doctor/patient relationships. Heart disease has been the leading cause of death of American women since 1908 but is misdiagnosed in women with alarming frequency. Breast cancer is another disease in which medicine staggers from one monstrosity to another. The notorious tamoxifen study, begun in 1992, is startling example:

> But just as critics feared, by early 1994, some two years into the five-year study, trouble was on the horizon. Data from another breast cancer trial being conducted by the National Surgical Adjuvant Breast and Bowel Project [NSABP] found that twenty-three women with breast cancer who were taking tamoxifen to prevent a recurrence had developed uterine cancer. Four of those women died from the disease. Amazingly, Bernard Fisher had known about two of the deaths as early as September 1993 but delayed reporting them to NCI officials until November, presumably because he was concerned about the bad publicity that would be generated. Even more outrageous, it wasn't until January 1994 that the healthy women participating in the breast cancer prevention trial were told of the deaths. Then in March, news broke about falsified data in the NSABP's lumpectomy trials, raising questions about the safety and efficacy of this surgical technique. Admitting its inability to monitor the quality of Bernard Fisher's research, in April the NCI temporarily halted recruitment in all fourteen NSABP studies, including the Breast Cancer Prevention Trial.[4]

Leslie Laurence and Beth Weinhouse, authors of *Outrageous Practices*, admit that the practice of conventional medicine "...to treat healthy women with a drug rather than investigating possible risk factors that are under their control, such as diet, seems ludicrous." But this is exactly what happens over and over. Breast-cancer activists have long stated that less money should be thrown at treatment and detection and more at finding the causes of the disease. Studies of dietary changes made by women never received funding from the National Cancer Institute. When heart disease was studied in men, however, dietary changes were considered entirely relevant. Laurence and Weinhouse conclude:

> Ultimately the message was that learning whether reducing dietary fat might prevent women from getting breast cancer was not im-

> portant. More precisely, encouraging women to eat a low-fat diet was not a potential moneymaker. But pouring federal funds into the search for new drugs, into high technology, that spelled patents and profits was. In the laboratory, with the test tubes and beakers and multi-million-dollar equipment, where the testosterone flowed, that's where real science happened. It was laughable to think that NCI, the quintessential old-boys' club, would study something as low tech as diet and breast cancer.

A later study that monitored the eating habits of almost ninety thousand nurses over an eight-year period found no correlation in breast cancer rates and their consumption of fat.[5]

The authors paint a similar picture when it comes to surgery on women. An all-or-nothing philosophy is responsible for thousands of hysterectomies, mastectomies, surgicalization of childbirth leading to cesarean section, episiotomies, and the sexy selling of cosmetic surgery.[6] According to *Outrageous Practices*, there are a staggering 550 thousand hysterectomies performed every year in the United States. Another example of gender lines within research and implementation of treatment is the popular hormone-replacement therapy to delay the onset of menopause. There are strong indicators that hormone-replacement therapy may have severe detrimental impacts ranging from accelerating the onset of osteoporosis to the great unknowns in the connection between hormone replacement and heart disease and its troublesome connection to breast cancer.[7] We should be alarmed. In spite of the disquieting lack of information, these products are fervently marketed, providing one more example where the medicalization of society becomes the prime causes for disease.

Science and commerce: an unholy alliance

The scientific-rational approach quickly spilled over into the areas of economics and commerce. Economy came to be defined as a disconnected, disassociated number of humans who were commercially active, selling property and services, buying goods, and so on. The principle of gravity was transposed into the miraculous guidance of the market. Market forces were attributed with human intelligence. Today the market-force superstition rises above morals and religion to become the one concept that almost everybody believes in. Divine right ultimately was replaced by market right.

These were indeed important yet ominous changes. At the time of a church-controlled worldview, accumulation of material goods, while certainly popular, was not yet the highest officially proclaimed goal. However, with rationalism and commerce soundly in place, the charging of interest became acceptable. Land that was once God-given now became a golden commodity and prospectors from the more industrialized European countries would venture around the globe to seek out and exploit nature's valuable resources.

All this rationalism and commerce resulted in enormous technological innovations, which made man feel as if he were manipulating reality and sitting, in the best tradition of Francis Bacon, on top of nature. But there were also voices of doubt. By 1905, Max Weber regretted the loss of spiritual richness that had given way to the rationalist ethic, and dryly summed up what he thought of modern man: "Specialists without spirit, sensualists without heart, this nothingness imagines that it has attained a level of civilization never before achieved."[8] These are the consequences of our familiar theme of disconnection from nature for the sake of commerce and consumer economics.

Now, in the late twentieth century, rationalism has produced frightening consequences. The elimination of soul and compassion in favor of an ice-cold economic rationalism has brought humanity to the brink of self-destruction by accepting gradual suicide so commerce can continue as usual. The societies of the Western world constantly invent new dehumanizing ways to perpetuate their denial while the developing countries suffer the consequences of the West's economic activities. The superstition of the infallibility of markets has been so ingrained in the consciousness of society that even the most horrific consequences are apathetically and mindlessly endured. The absolutely infallible authority of market is accepted without any explanation or proof. This brainwashing has worked beyond belief.

These peculiarities should be kept in mind to evaluate the scientific merit of conventional medicine correctly. Conventional wisdom holds that medical science understands the cause of disease, especially the cause of infectious disease. According to this understanding, pathogenic germs *are* the cause of infectious disease. The conventional procedure is to identify the disease first (diagnose), attaching a name to it and then treating it. Often, "treatment" means killing the implicated microorganisms or suppressing the predominant symptoms of the disease through the prescription of drugs. Because the scientific process needs to verify and produce results, it puts the disease at the center of attention—germs can be killed and symptoms alleviated in reproducible experiments. But people are individuals and the unique conditions of their health and lives cannot be standardized. People are unruly objects for medical research. Conventional methodology must concentrate on aspects that can supposedly be objectified, so it focuses on symptom, disease, and the specific germs or agents causing the disease. All factors relating to the unique constitution of a patient—immune status, emotional stability, state of happiness, family, and so on—are considered secondary. No *thinking* medical practitioner would truly believe these human factors are of minor importance, but because the whole system depends on making everything objective, there is no space for the subjective elements of human life. How incredibly deeply this mechanistic view of disease and healing has been ingrained in the collective consciousness is reflected in the political discussion about the costs and affordability of health care. Only conventional medicine has the degree of scientific basis and thus merits tax or insurance dollars. We are led to believe that alternative approaches are soft-core methods appropriate for lesser problems, and *real* medicine must be sought when the problems (diseases) become more serious and their treatments more expensive. As an automatic consequence of our economic system, treatments for serious conditions are expected to be expensive. A cheap cure for a serious disease severely overchallenges the imagination. This is reinforced by the press on almost any given day by editorial pieces compliantly reporting scientific breakthroughs that will cure today's incurable diseases tomorrow. Armed with enough scientific research, we are supposed to believe that every medical puzzle is solvable.

The antibiotics crisis

There is conclusive evidence on the destructive consequences of the overuse of antibiotics (and also how to avoid it).[9] Antibiotic pressure on an organism can be a cofactor in immune deficiency conditions. Antibiotics were originally prescribed to fight bacterial diseases. But once these drugs became major moneymakers, their marketing took on a life of its own. Economic interest dictates finding more uses for a product that is already selling well, because sales increase without new development costs. Research to find additional uses for products is eagerly sponsored and eventually research and sales create a new reality. Unaware of the link to mass destruction of their immune systems, an unsuspecting generation upped its antibiotic intake.

Antibiotics taken by small children often create the diseases they aim to cure. Premature antibiotic use during the onset of a childhood disease will deprive the immune system of the opportunity to interact with the pathogen.[10] An inactivated immune system does not learn to recognize intruding microorganisms, nor does it learn to build antibodies. The result? A child will quickly relapse with the same disease and the cycle repeats. A recurring disease becomes chronic and leads to an overall debilitation of the body.

Another potentially even greater problem is the seemingly unstoppable advance of resistant bacteria. Bacteria, resistant to most or all of the known antibiotics, are menacing hospitals and their patients. The development of these "super germs" was brought on by the reckless use of antibiotics in the meat industry as well as their overprescription by doctors. In his sanely radical *Spontaneous Heal-*

ing, Andrew Weil comments: "Doctors must bear much of the responsibility for getting us into our growing predicament with aggressive bacteria; by over-prescribing and mis-prescribing antibiotics, they have brought on the coming catastrophe."[11]

Antibiotics are still widely prescribed by doctors for viral conditions such as the common cold or the flu despite the fact that they are not effective in these cases. The depth of the conditioning becomes obvious when antibiotics display placebo effects.

Workers in an office struggle with the flu for a week or two and, at some point, a few take antibiotics.

Outcome 1: No obvious differences are observed between those who take the antibiotics and those who don't. The flu comes and goes.

Outcome 2: Some of those who took antibiotics recover quickly. A typical belief is that the antibiotics ultimately cured the flu.

Outcome 2 is extremely puzzling. *Influenza is a viral infection and antibiotics are not effective against viruses*. Still, these individuals claim that they worked. There are two possible explanations: 1. The immune status of some individuals is so compromised from antibiotics overuse or other causes that a flu virus will automatically trigger bacterial secondary infections of such severity that relief from the accompanying symptoms is perceived as the antibiotics being effective against the flu itself. 2. Our deep conditioning to believe in the effectiveness of antibiotics triggers improvement. The antibiotics were a placebo!

The antibiotics crisis is an example of the fact that commerce is not concerned about the consequences it creates for human life. All aspects of modern existence are penetrated by the goal to maximize profits. Sadly, this has been most successful in medicine.[12]

Approximately two decades ago the projections for worldwide sales of pharmaceuticals for the year 2000 were estimated to reach about $250 billion. This number was a *gross* underestimation; the health-care industry currently grosses almost a thousand billion dollars and the biggest-selling pharmaceutical drugs each generate one billion dollars annually in the United States alone. Potential pharmacological breakthroughs generate corresponding changes in stock prices and make headlines in the business sections. The profit motive permeates the medical world completely.

As a result, diseases are essentially classified according to the availability of drugs, which are the only form of therapy that can be produced on an industrial scale. The drug companies have an ideal partner in scientific medicine, which ignores (for the most part) social and psychological causes of disease. The mechanic "physician" is offered a tool that can be reproduced without limit.

Sponsoring reality

Competing for money became the ultimate scientific rationale. Some, especially elite universities after World War II, led the way to make this rational economic worldview—simplistically called greed—their modus operandi.[13] Research was routinely conducted in those areas for which corporate sponsorship or government-commissioned defense research filled the coffers of the university. The topics that brought in the money were the ones eagerly researched. The more money, the more elite the university. At a time when money was the measure of everything, the fact that the universities lost their scientific independence as a result of these practices was not even worth lamenting. Actually, universities did not *lose* their independence, they were eager to give it up in exchange for dollars.

The way science is manufactured has changed drastically over the last fifty years. Before World War II, American universities defined themselves mainly in terms of their independence, their *isolation,* from the doings of government and commerce. By the early sixties the country's big and prestigious universities obtained nearly 50 percent of their operating budgets from federal research grants and were establishing more special schools and institutes with the aim of collecting money from foundations and corporate donors. They educated experts in the political economies of communist countries, and physicists were drawn into the development of miracle weapons. Eventually, the hard sciences were drawn into researching how to fight the cold war. Next were the social scientists needed for the psychological war and the propaganda campaigns that accompanied the arms race. Researchers gave in to the call of patriotism and bigger budgets despite concerns over losing academic freedom and traditional values of unbiased inquiry. But there was no concern about losing academic independence; Stanford University is one example of a campus eager to become a partner with government, industry, and foundation patrons. The traditional goals of educating undergraduates and supporting diverse but often impractical fundamental research disappeared. Departments reduced teaching in favor of research and publication, which created a new entrepreneurial and star-based hierarchy based on access to money rather than seniority or scientific achievements. Fields deemed unimportant (without sponsors) were terminated. Stanford University's School of Mineral Sciences was forced to eliminate smaller classes and instead focus on metallurgy and materials that science needed for military and commercial electronics, to the exclusion of other fields. The manner in which Stanford University integrated itself into a network of private industry and government sponsors turned its ideals upside down and banished critical thought. This has immediate consequences for the alleged validity and objectivity of medical research. Uncritically, we might assume that medical research emanates from the desire to seek the truth. In the contemporary university nothing could be further from the truth. What happened at Stanford University is typical for all of academia in the last decades.

Because essential oils are not patentable and profit expectations are zero, there is no corporate sponsorship and therefore there is hardly any science. Essential oils are no longer researched at university level, which therefore creates the perception that these medicines are weak, useless, or ineffective. This is a direct outcome of the sellout of academia to corporate sponsorship. This has gone to the extreme that research into medicinal plants has left the North

American continent and is now favored in countries such as Brazil and Turkey. This is the most important fact to be remembered when the scientific merits of alternative therapies are discussed.[14]

"Existing knowledge" is no longer generated by impartial, unbiased research, but almost exclusively through corporate funding. Insidiously, science has been denigrated to become a tool for the fabrication of a reality planned by corporate strategists. Not just the uninformed fall victim to this situation; it also permeates the medical profession. In Candace Pert's *Molecules of Emotion*, the author describes the situation: "Why aren't doctors making available the natural, plant-derived forms of estrogen and progesterone, substances that are known to have fewer side effects than their laboratory-produced analogs? The answer reflects the economics of medicine: Since the natural substances are not patentable, there is no incentive for drug companies to study their benefits, and so the vast majority of M.D.s, who get their information about drugs from the drug companies, don't even know about them!"

Essential oils: nonpatentable, noncorporate

There is no incentive for corporations to fund essential-oils research. As they are in the public domain, it is not possible to patent essential oils, so corporations can not profit from control of the product. Novel *uses* of oils could actually be protected by patents. But profiting from a use, rather than controlling the substance itself, is cumbersome. Besides, aromatherapy is too small a market. Since virtually no current research exists, aromatherapy's claims rest on traditional and anecdotal lore. The reality of aromatherapy is therefore only partly defined by science. Integrating aspects of live and healing aromatherapy is unavailable to the material world of science. An example of how this system works may be seen in the case of tea tree oil, *Melaleuca alternifolia*. As soon as commercial prospects increased for this versatile and effective botanical, the number of studies multiplied.[15] There had been a modest number of studies in Australia by the first half of this century, but as tea tree oil grew in commercially relevant proportions, fairly detailed studies on its effects, composition, harvesting, and chemotypes emerged. Again, what we know or accept as truth is directly related to the size of commerce of the research object. If we maintain that language creates reality, one could even fall into a perception that things or concepts do not exist before there is money to purchase an inquiry into their reality.

Another problem is that too often the attempts of self-appointed guardians of scientific accuracy in aromatherapy to demonstrate the availability or the lack of evidence are quite superficial. In the past, traditional scientific procedure began with an investigation and a thorough assessment of the existing literature, the existing body of knowledge. It may be a sign of our times that a short attention span is also reflected in the work of contemporary scientists who find neither the time nor the energy to look at the available evidence before they set out to conduct more research or formulate their statements. As a consequence, abundant scientific documentation on the pharmacology of essential oils, especially in German and French scientific literature, is overlooked.[16]

The inconvenience of having many of the works published only in the French or German language translates into the denial of the existence of these works. Because there is no truly academic foundation for aromatherapy, especially in our English-speaking environment, some who claim to be "scientific" get away with something more aptly called xenophobic indolence, the utter disregard for results published in other languages. Sadly, what in truth is a flawed scientific procedure is presented as objective truth. Some protest that many of these studies are dated and therefore potentially obsolete, but this ignores the fact that observed empirical effects are as true today as they ever were. Empirical observations stand regardless of the changing fashion of analytical gadgetry.

A substantial body of scientific studies already exists, which provides a perfect pharmacological rationale for many of the applications of essential oils. If anyone had the desire to search the relevant databases for published studies on essential-oil pharmacology, he or she would find that much of what is claimed is already scientifically proven. It is virtually inconceivable for academic scientists trying to conduct clean and credible research to suggest that there is no scientific corroboration for the effects of aromatherapy. Ignoring it amounts to bad science.

An examination of the blessings progress has brought is a scary enterprise. Things should be marvelous after so much progress, but instead there is a reactionary desire to return to the "good old days," especially in the political arena. Why have ever-newer technologies not created the promised paradise for society and produced solutions for the most important medical problems? The answer lies in the choice the economic system has made for us, which is to devalue human life in favor of corporate profits.

Medical nemesis

In the medical world, this finds its depressing expression in the well-documented rituals the pharmaceutical industry performs to either bring questionable drugs to market or to keep them in distribution even if hazards have been proven.[17] Patients' welfare takes a back seat to uninterrupted sales. People suffering from "civilization diseases," such as cancer and the various autoimmune diseases—are paying the price for the choices made in the name of commerce, progress, and pharmacology. The consequences of society-wide antibiotics overuse, environmental degradation, industrial pollution, and the toxic ideas that spew out of our many channels of media and entertainment have all taken a toll on the integrity of our immune systems. Oddly enough, corporate structure is similar to the current medical paradigm, with its prescribed hierarchy of human relations resembling a steep and narrowing pyramid with the maximum wealth on top and a teeming lower tier of expendable and powerless labor below. Drug development is entirely profit-driven and will orient itself to the size and affluence of an expected target group. What this means is that a few will gain huge profits from new drug development while the rest of us take Prozac.

The latest success of the pharmaceutical industry's quest for bigger sales is the development of new drugs that large parts of the population are told to take continuously. Drugs like Tamoxifen are prescribed with orders to be taken continuously by women who are deemed to have an increased risk of breast cancer. Prozac and Viagra have ushered in the era of "lifestyle" drugs. Taking such drugs continuously, by large segments of the population, obviously increases sales and profitability for the large corporations. The concept behind this is the same as the one that helped psychology become a part of mass culture—successfully obscuring the differences between being diseased and being healthy. If the healthy part of the population can be treated too, sales skyrocket. The truly diseased part of the population may not be financially exploitable, so convincing the healthy and wealthy part of population of the need for drugs ensures the continued growth of sales.

In their drive for economic efficiency, pharmaceutical companies have no choice but to focus all research, development, and policy on one single goal: maximum profit. Conversely, holistic healing systems would be serving the long-term interest of everyone and make the world more inhabitable, not less. But corporate entertainment presents us with emotionally charged hospital emergency-room dramas, making sure that such concepts remain far from public consciousness.

The ultimate conditions resulting from technology and the irrepressible rise of the highly paid expert were described by Ivan Illich more than twenty years ago: if healing is left to the self-serving powers of commercialized science, the resulting drugs and prescription medications will themselves become the major cause of disease, creating an apocalyptic reality of medical nemesis. Illich describes the crippling consequences of handing over responsibility to the experts of techno medicine:

> With the transformation of the doctor from an artisan exercising a skill on a personally known individual into a technician applying

> scientific rules to classes of patients, malpractice acquired an anonymous, almost respectable status. What had formerly been considered an abuse of confidence and a moral fault can now be rationalized into the occasional breakdown of equipment and operators. In a complex technological hospital negligence becomes "random human error" or "system break-down," callousness becomes "scientific" detachment, and incompetence becomes a lack of specialized equipment.[18]

While the medical system pretends to serve the general population, it is truly only accountable to shareholders, not the patients.[19] To perpetrate this situation, the concept of responsibility for questions of medicine has been turned entirely upside down when it comes to laypeople. Patients are supposedly acting responsibly when they surrender themselves to the medical deities. Obviously this arrangement does not, as ancient or modern holistic healing does, take any responsibility for the drugs or treatments prescribed. (Some early practitioners of medicine forfeited payment if their patient was not cured.) Instead, conventional medical treatments follow specific protocols by which the drugs are supposed to "work." If they fail, it is the insufficiency of progress or the pill itself, rather than the failure of the drug company or the doctor's recommendations.

In the end, the medical system provides a service according to a set procedure and is not responsible for anything. And nothing is more demoralizing than to be controlled by those who do not take responsibility, because it prevents the patient, who is subject to this control, from helping him- or herself.

It is exactly in the commercial interest of the pharmaceutical system to perpetuate this situation. Decades ago, Franklin D. Roosevelt foresaw this and warned repeatedly that technology without moral controls would be a "ruthless master of mankind." Freedom is not safe if private power is tolerated and grows until it becomes stronger than the democratic state. In his conclusion this was, in fact, fascism.[20]

How could this happen?

The fact that we are so helpless over the impositions of the medical system is that little or no thought is given to how the beliefs we hold ever came into being. We may think that they are the normal consequence of evolution or progress. Actually, many of these concepts are perfectly unnatural. Visiters from developing countries are often painfully aware of our distance from nature. In the extrapolated consequence of the scientific revolution, the body came to be seen as a machine with more or less effectively greased single parts. Planet Earth was reduced to an exploitable, natural resource and, with commercial air travel becoming more affordable, we forgot where we once belonged. This disassociation is obvious in the way we allow ourselves to be exclusively ruled by our minds, the way we trash our sexual needs, and the extent of our desire for individual advancement. If it were possible, it seems we would all be believers in a form of enlightenment far removed from bodies or sex. Merely having a body has become a central embarrassment. Instead, the current seductive trend is to sit in front of twenty-four-inch, full-color, high-resolution screens to communicate with other bodyless people. We can now work, play, shop, read, bank, and chat electronically in front of this illuminated screen. Our senses of smell and touch become marginal. Primary realities like pain and illness have no reason; symptoms have no purpose but are medicated away with brightly colored pills. We forget that we have bodies (except for shaping them) and that human life used to be and still should be treated with respect. It is only if, after a lifetime of avoiding our bodies and basic humanistic concepts, we have to meet face to face with an illness that refuses to be managed away with a course of antibiotics that we discover our souls again. Illness teaches us lessons that high-tech pharmacology and formal education have overlooked: we are mortal, we have bodies that register sensations, and we interact with our earthly environment. Indeed, we might discover many of the things that are truly important by paying more attention to these bodily reactions, to the sensations we perceive.

A human direction for science

The point is not to remove scientific and technological advantages that humanity has gained. The direction of scientific research needs to be considered carefully, however. Where is it going, what is it doing, and what does it mean for the future of humans? This is exemplified with the human genome project, the gargantuan project (three billion dollars) in which the National Center for Human Genome Research (a branch of NIH) set out to locate all the genes within the human body by the year 2005. Schumacher, in *Small Is Beautiful,* writes, "We cannot leave this to the scientists alone." Einstein rightfully observed that almost all scientists are economically completely dependent and the number of scientists who possess a sense of social responsibility is so small that they cannot determine the direction of research. The later dictum applies, no doubt, to most or all medical specialists and the task therefore falls to the intelligent laymen. This view seems to be supported by even the most ardent advocates of scientific developments.

In *Visions,* an insightful book how science will revolutionize the twenty-first century, Michio Kaku writes about the fabulous future advances science will make unless nuclear war, the outbreak of a deadly epidemic, or an environmental collapse will spoil it all. One is left to assume that such potential catastrophes are not brought on by science but by politicians or forms of human irresponsibility: "Unfortunately resistant bacteria were allowed to flourish due to foolish short sighted health policies." Or, "As the pace of industrialization speeds up we expect more emergent and resistant diseases to appear" and "For example, Legionnaires' disease, toxic shock syndrome and Lyme disease are examples of disease which have spread as a consequence of modernization within the United States." Carefully discussed are the deeply troubling issues of what ethical ramifications future research will present. The awesome scientific knowledge that will be unveiled early in the next century must be tempered by the enormous ethical, social, and political questions that it raises. Interesting parallels between nuclear energy and bioengineering are drawn. However precise and honest the reporting, the potential that maybe science itself could be at the core of the problem is not mentioned. Instead, lack of democratic discussion is given as the cause for the fact that the United States is now faced with seventeen leaking nuclear-weapons dumps that may cost upward of 500 billion dollars to clean up. The human cost can not be estimated.

Visions does not attempt to decide whether democratic states, scientists, or business leaders should take responsibility for the outcome of whatever the next experiment is. Behavior based on nature, including alternative medical modalities, provides solace in the fact that products of the living earth pose none of these questions, as opposed to medical developments such as chemotherapy that generate huge ethical problems.

In *Visions,* the head of the human genome project states, "Genetic information itself is not going to hurt the public. What could hurt the public is existing social structures, policies and prejudices against which information can ricochet. We need genetic information right now in order to make better choices so we can live better lives. We need the improved treatments that will eventually be developed using genetic information. So, I think the answer is certainly not to slow down the advancing science, but to try, somehow to make the social system more accommodating to new knowledge."[21] The hierarchy is clear: advancing science first, humans second. Later in the book, a technology-assessment report is quoted: "Applicants for insurance plans are already being asked to provide information to prospective insurers related to genetic conditions like sickle cell anemia." Some experts fear individual policies will become increasingly difficult to acquire as more genetic screening tests become available. Implicit is that the financial success of the insurance company is the highest value. Everything else, including people who search for policies, is secondary.

There is no reason to assume that the scientific and technological spiral in the current economic system will ever stop. Money has the power to direct science to where it sees profits, and it will do so regardless of any destruction this might create. *Visions* concedes that these dynamics will continue: "Unfortunately, biological warfare has a long and ugly history." In light of this the opinion of a legislative supporter of the genome project sounds self-defeating: "If you believe that one the strongest mandates of human kind is to pursue ways to alleviate human suffering, you really cannot be against this research. But it is knowledge. It is not good or evil. It is just knowledge." And a final note from this book: "In the future society must be wary of those who would use the benefits of the genetic revolution to further their own social agenda." To cement power through knowledge, to cement the superiority of the technological way of life; to assure even bigger profits for health insurers (who are one of the forces behind this research)? What Kaku's book cannot hide is that money rules, that what *can* be done will be done.

Unnecessarily inflicted human suffering stops with the termination of the research on how to make people suffer. Low-tech modalities do not require any future research—they can be explored by humans through regular experiential processes. Just imagine the grizzly consequences of our scientific frenzy, and you'll gain faith in less-spectacular options. Relying on natural methods makes for a more secure well-being. That the scientific-technological process often leaves humans empty is also recognized in countries of the developing world, where the consequences are often felt even more painfully.

In an essay called "Reductionist Science as Epistemological Violence," the Indian physicist Vandana Shiva deplores the sweeping dismissal of local knowledge—about agriculture, for instance—that is enforced by the scientific arrogance inherent in the modern model of development.[22] She calls the often highly incentive implementation of technologies that might be useful in one society but largely counterproductive in another "structural violence." She notes a reduction in the range of acceptable knowledge not only among the "alleged beneficiaries," but also among scientists themselves. In "Science as a Reason of the State," Ashis Nandy asserts that the legitimacy of the post-colonial state rests on the unrestrained authority of scientists, national security experts, and development specialists. He asks, "Can one not go beyond shedding tears copiously over the misuse of modern science by wicked politicians, militarists and multinational corporations, and scrutinize the popular culture and philosophy of modern science? May the sources of violence not lie partly in the nature of science itself? Is there something in modern science itself which makes it a human enterprise particularly open to co-optation by the powerful and wealthy?" Like other critics of modernity, these Indian analysts do not advocate a rejection of modern science but a creative option that would integrate significant knowledge from premodern, nonmodern, and postmodern science as well.

Similar if not more radical ideas are part of an effort to "decolonize" Peru's culture. The goal is to become "non-subjects" by thinking and acting in ways that are far removed from those of the modern West, and to honor the native worldview as a legitimate frame of reference from which dialogue with other cultures may take place. *Proyecto Andino de Technologias Campesinas* (PRATEC) of the Peruvian Andes is devoted to research and writing about Andean technologies, knowledge, and worldview. Its members advocate neither a cultural fundamentalism nor a "hybrid" culture of modern and nonmodern but rather a "cultural affirmation" that questions the evolutionary inevitability of "progress" and modernization. At the heart of their dialogue is a spiritual conversation of remarkable openness and attentiveness to all beings of earth's communities—rivers, animals, and other peoples.

Vaclav Havel, Czech president and author, expresses the growing concern with eloquence: "We may know immeasurably more about the universe than our ancestors did, and yet increasingly it seems they knew something more essential about it than we do—something that escapes us. The same is true of our own human nature. The more thoroughly our organs, their functions, internal structures and the biochemical reactions that occur within them are described, the more we fail to grasp the spirit, purpose, and meaning of the system they co-create and which we experience as our unique self."

"It is the weight not the number of experiments that is to be regarded."
—Isaac Newton

SIX

Science and Plant Intelligence

The preceding chapters discussed historical and philosophical concepts behind the interaction of plants, humans, and aromatic substances. Aromatherapy also benefits from the fascinating evidence the scientific method has contributed to our knowledge of aromatic substances. This happened mostly as a result of disciplines other than aromatherapy researching essential oils.

Unraveling the secrets of essential oils

In the late nineteenth century, essential-oil production in the town of Grasse, in the south of France, had been developed to near perfection, but virtually nothing was known about the actual composition of the oils.[1] The first acknowledgment of the different components in essential oils was made by old hands working in Grasse (the town has been making perfumes since the fifteenth century). They had recognized the similarities between terpene-rich essential oils and turpentine, and sesquiterpene-rich essential oils and gurjum balsam. When turpentine and gurjum were used as adulterants they were described in very evocative terms in the dialect of the province: *La Musica* and *Lou Faber*.

A more detailed understanding of the actual chemical composition of essential oils began with the work of chemist Otto Wallach between the years 1880 and 1914. Otto Wallach was an assistant of the eminent F.A. Kekulé, the first to accurately describe the chemical structure of the benzene molecule. His interest was triggered when he found some old, abandoned essential-oil bottles in Kekulé's laboratory.[2]

In Wallach's day it was known that hydrocarbons existed with the molecular formula $C_{10} H_{16}$. Because of their presence in turpentine, Kekulé had named them terpenes. At that time, deriving a summary formula of a molecule showing how many of each atom were present was the extent of the possible characterization (structural formulas were only to arise later), and chemists were facing enormous difficulties in their attempts to elucidate the composition of these molecules. Substances with similar formulas, namely $C_{10} H_{16}O$ and $C_{10} H_{18}O$, were obviously related to the terpenes and identified by the generic name "camphor." The prototype of this group of compounds was camphor itself, which was known since antiquity in the Orient and since the eleventh century in Europe. Terpenes were considered difficult to study because the differences that distinguished them were so minuscule. Kekulé always preferred to study the more clearly separated benzene-related molecules and considered research of essential-oil components not a tempting venture.

Based on their botanical sources, terpenes were characterized by many different names even though they were often chemically identical. Wallach's plan was to identify basic properties that would distinguish the individual chemicals, to study any pure chemicals that could be isolated, and to understand their precise chemical constitutions. In 1884 Wallach succeeded in showing that several terpenes described under different names were in fact the same substance. In 1891 he established a list of nine different terpenes that he could characterize. These were pinene, camphene, fenchene, limonene, dipentene, phellandrene, terpinolene, and sylvestrene. (Sylvestrene was actually an artifact of distillation stemming from the terpene carene.) Subsequently, he recognized that what he had originally considered to be the single substances pinene, terpinene, and phellandrene were actually mixtures of isomers. Wallach separated these substances by systematic fractional distillation. To find clues about their chemical composition, he let the separated substances react with inorganic reagents and characterized the resulting (often crystallizable) products. From 1884 to 1914 he wrote 180 papers that were later assembled into a single book called *Terpene and Camphor.* He had realized that these compounds must be constructed from isoprene units. Thirty years later, in 1947, Robinson was awarded the Nobel prize in chemistry for showing that the buildup of terpenes occurred through connecting isoprene molecules in a head-to-tail fashion. Wallach's work was the starting point of essential-oil chemistry and shaped many aspects of organic chemistry as a whole. He received the Nobel prize in chemistry in 1910. Another chemist, Adolf von Bayer, pioneered the development of structural formulas of terpene molecules. With Wallach, he devoted considerable work toward elucidating the structural formula of pinene. The pinene molecule includes, as Wallach and von Baeyer had suspected, a four carbon ring structure. The structure of alpha-pinene as it is currently accepted was first proposed by Wagner in 1894 and was based on the rigid experimentation of von Baeyer between the years 1896 and 1907. Von Baeyer pioneered the study of the symmetry of molecules and specifically the implications of atoms being attached in different positions on a ring system. His considerations led to the development of stereo chemistry. There were many other chemists who contributed to the progress of the field: Thiemann, Semmler, Wagner, Gildemeister, Hoffmann, and, in France, Grignard and Dupont. From 1920 forward, Ruzicka of Switzerland became the real successor to Wallach's work. Despite this considerable effort, only a small number of monoterpenes were well known at the beginning of the twentieth century. The first correct chemical structure of a sesquiterpene, beta-santalene, was determined by Semmler in 1910. Three years later the chemical structure of a second sesquiterpene, farnesene, was determined. Knowledge about the other large group of essential oil constituents, the phenylpropanoids, had come somewhat earlier, probably due to their less complex nature. The summary formula of cinnamic aldehyde was established by Dumas and Pilligot in 1834, but its exact structure was only determined in 1866 by Erlenmeyer.

The structure elucidation of musk odorants, large ring systems consisting of up to fifteen carbon atoms, earned Ruzicka the Nobel prize in 1939. Shortly after World War II, two major encyclopedias on every aspect of essential oil chemistry, cultivation, and pharmacology were published: the *Guenther* volumes and the *Gildemeister & Hoffmann*.[3] Analytical methods to determine the structure of essential-oil molecules were still based on carrying out actual chemical reactions and obtaining clues from the resulting products and the conversions that had taken place.

Next came instrumental analysis. Before World War II, chemists had to separate the components of essential oils by tedious distillation processes. Today, improved chromatographic methods, liquid chromatography, and high-pressure liquid chromatography make it much easier to separate an essential oil into its (often) hundreds of components. The spectroscopic methods of studying the molecular structure of the isolated substances became better too.[4] Spectroscopic methods measure physical qualities of a given molecule, which allows for conclusions about its molecular structure. With infrared spectroscopy, ultraviolet spectroscopy, nuclear-magnetic-resonance spectroscopy, and the perfection of mass-spectroscopy, determining accurate molecular structures for many of the more elusive essential-oil components became routine. The structure of highly odor-effective components such as damascenone and rose-oxide in rose or the jasmonates in jasmine would never have been revealed without the help of these methods.

In 1969 a group of researchers, F. W. Hefendal, Karl-Heinz Kubeczka, J. Carlsen, and A. Baerheim-Svendsen, who had made essential oils their main topic, gathered for the first time for what was then modestly called a "workshop" to discuss their mutual work. These meetings developed into the International Symposium on Essential Oils, and Professor Karl-Heinz Kubeczka, among others, must be credited with creating this premier forum for the publication of the latest research on the chemistry of essential oils.[5] In the early years the application of new and improved chromatographic and spectroscopic methods to elucidate the composition of essential oils was a major focus. Some outstanding contributions during the beginning years held great interest for the purposes of aromatherapy: "Distribution of Essential Oils in the Plant Kingdom," by R. Hegnauer, "Possibilities of Quality Determination of Medicinally Used Essential Oils," by Kubeczka, and "Processes in an Essential Oil Glandular Cell of a Plant," by G. Heinrich.[6] Papers on the optimization of gas chromatographic and mass-spectroscopic methods for the analysis of essential oils created the basis for today's standard analytic procedures; two fine examples are "Systematic Identification and Structure Elucidation of Sesquiterpenes," by G. Rücker, and an overview on the analysis of components occurring in German chamomile by H. Schilcher.[7] A high point of these congresses was reached with the 16th International Symposium, which celebrated the seventy-fifth anniversary of Otto Wallach's Nobel prize.[8] The compositions of bay laurel oil and many other plants were reported.[9] A particularly interesting paper on isolation and synthesis of compounds from the essential oil of *Helichrysum italicum* was presented by T. Weyerstahl and coworkers.[10] One detailed paper described the action of terpenoid components such as menthol, camphor, eugenol, and thymol on the oxygen metabolism in the cell membrane.[11]

A short history of essential-oil pharmacology

Inquiry into the pharmacological aspects of essential oils against infectious diseases represents by far the most research involving essential oils, which perhaps reflects this century's preoccupation with infection. Additionally, the psychological effects of essential oils began to move into focus. After World War II, the division of labor peaked and resulting health conditions such as nervousness, fatigue, anxiety, and depression set in.

Early scientific inquiry into the pharmacological properties of essential oils is impressively represented in Gattefossé's *Aromather-*

apie. More than 300 studies, conducted between the end of the nineteenth century and the early 1930s, are referenced. While some of these studies are between seventy and a hundred years old, they were conducted with clear, scientific methodology and form the basis of our scientific understanding of the properties of essential-oil components.

Antimicrobial effects of essential oils

This line of research began with some classical studies at the Pasteur Institute. Microbes were isolated in a culture medium and then subjected to an essential oil. If the essential oil effectively killed or inhibited the bacterium, the result was considered positive.

Table 6.1: Selected historical studies on essential oils and their anti-infectious effects

1881:	Koch studied the bactericidal action of turpentine essence on anthrax spores
1887:	Chamberland studied the activity of the essences of oregano, cinnamon, and clove on bacillus anthracis.
1910:	Martindale showed that the essential oil of oregano is the strongest plant-derived antiseptic known to date. Oregano is twenty-five to seventy-six times more active than isolated phenol on the colibacillus.

The superior ability of essential oils to disinfect room air was demonstrated in 1956.[12] In 1973 Hildebert Wagner demonstrated that a mix of common essential-oil constituents had a broader spectrum of action than broad spectrum antibiotics, especially with respect to bacteria implicated in upper respiratory infections.[13] At the same time, effectiveness against *Candida albicans* by mountain savory and other essential oils was demonstrated.[14] A climax was reached with broad-based assessment of antibacterial and antifungal properties with the aromatogram technique (described in part III), and the results showed oregano, thyme, clove, cinnamon, and tea tree to have the broadest overall spectrum of action.[15]

Table 6.2: Modern works: highlights

1949–1950:	Schroeder and Messing developed a technique that later became the aromatogram.
1954–1956:	Kellner and Kobert published a study on the action of 175 essential oils against eight airborne bacteria and fungi. They identified a group of twenty-one particularly active oils, including Spanish oregano.
1960:	Maruzzella demonstrated antibacterial and antifungal effects of hundreds of aromatic compounds.
1969:	M. Girault used the aromatogram technique to develop effective essential oil treatments for the specific flora of each patient.
1972:	H. Audhoui, P. Belaiche, J. Bourgeon, P. Duraffourd, C. Duraffourd, M. Girault, and J. C. Lapraz employed the aromatogram technique to develop treatments for a broad range of infectious illnesses. Forty essences and one tincture were studied.
1973:	Jacques Pellecuer reestablished the antibacterial and antifungal actions of the Mediterranean *labiatae*, rosemary and thyme, and the phenomenal effectiveness of *Satureja montana*.
1973:	Wagner and Sprinkmeyer demonstrated an essential-oil mix to have broader activity than broad spectrum antibiotics.
1987:	Deininger and Lembke demonstrated antiviral activity of essential oils and their isolated components.

Essential oils and the autonomic nervous system

At the same time Belaiche was conducting his research, essential oils, terpenes, and phenylpropanoids were also researched rather thoroughly in Germany in three major areas: sedative and spasmolytic effects, clinical studies demonstrating effectiveness for problems caused by autonomic nervous system imbalances, and in vitro and in vivo demonstration of the antiviral properties of essential oils.

The research was conducted to gain scientific proof of the many beneficial effects of a product composed entirely of distillates of aromatic plants available in Germany: Klosterfrau Melissengeist

(KMG). Its 170-year-old formula enjoys a continuing commercial success. Melissengeist's composition reaches back to Paracelsus and contains the empirically known effects of melissa and other essential-oil plants. The main components of Klosterfrau Melissengeist are frequently encountered mono- and sesquiterpenes and phenylpropanoids: limonene, gingiberine, eugenol, citral, citronellol, eugenyl acetate, borneol, cinnamic aldehyde, linalyl acetate, geraniol, cineole, and caryophyllene.

Table 6.3: Components of KMG

The product is an alcoholic co-distillate of:		
Folia melissae	*Rhizoma helenii*	*Radix angelicae*
Flores caryophylli	*Rhizoma galangae*	*Radix gentianae*
Rhizoma zingiberis	*Fructus piperis nigri*	

Through an effective coalition of university research and clinical evaluation of KMG, solid and convincing data on the effectiveness of essential oils was accumulated.[16] These studies are highly relevant for aromatherapy because the studied components are commonly found in many different essential oils and are representative for all chemical families encountered in essential oils.[17] Results for the alcohol geraniol are valid regardless of whether it is encountered in geranium or in palmarosa oil. Linalyl acetate displays its properties whether it's encountered in lavender, clary sage, or even in the linalool type of thyme or in petitgrain.

Sedatives and spasmolytics

In 1973 Wagner and Sprinkmeyer showed that all the tested substances of the KMG mixture have very good sedative properties. Most effective were linalool and eugenol. Most of the components showed their highest effectiveness at rather low concentrations, one milligram per one kilogram of body weight. Increasing the dosage often led to a decreased effect. The authors speculated that this was due to the inactivation of terpene receptors by larger dosages of terpenes. All of the tested compounds showed spasmolytic effects and eugenol and eugenyl acetate showed very strong inhibitory effects for contractions, equally effective as the clinical benchmark papaverin.[18] Antibacterial and bacteriostatic effectiveness of the KMG combination were assessed. The results showed that the combination had an extraordinarily broad spectrum of effectiveness against all of the tested bacteria, particularly those implicated in upper respiratory conditions. The authors concluded that the activity was broader than that of broad spectrum antibiotics, especially with respect to microorganisms occurring in respiratory diseases. In an interesting aside, the authors observed that synthetically derived specimens had lesser effects than the natural terpenes.

Autonomic nervous system imbalances

Imbalances of the autonomic nervous system do not appear to be a recognized condition in North American medicine and, according to Andrew Weil, practically do not even exist in the medical vocabulary! In Japan and Germany, two industrial societies with virtually identical industrial ills, "vegetative dystony" is the term used to describe this imbalance and the accompanying symptoms. Manifestations of autonomic nervous system imbalance are common symptoms such as headaches, hot flashes, irregular heartbeat, nervousness, depression, anxiety, and many similar symptomatic pictures.

Many common conditions in Western industrial societies are the consequence of autonomic nervous system imbalances. They originate from the conditions of modernity and urban technological lifestyles. Job-related stress, time pressure, environmental toxins, the frustrations of being forced to work in degrading jobs and the resulting alienation—a consequence of modern-day, money-chasing, technology-dependent lifestyles—as well as swallowing down fast food at red lights, subordinating family to economics, and insufficient relaxation can all be at the root of autonomic nervous system imbalance.

Clinical double-blind studies prove the ability of essential oils to alleviate many civilization diseases originating from autonomic nervous system imbalances. This therapeutic aspect of essential oils cannot be overestimated.[19] If the named conditions go untreated or if the conditions that lead to their onset are allowed to persist they will ultimately result in severe physical illnesses. As we age, these initially rather manageable conditions turn into irreversible, chronic civilization diseases. Preventing the onset and development of these grave consequences of decades under stress is possible with the help of essential oils. To some degree this allows us to stay healthy while living under the imposed condition of undesirable lifestyles. Profoundly noticeable is the fact that the use of essential oils—whether for relaxing baths, to maintain a healthy gastrointestinal tract, or to avoid antibiotics—minimizes the prechronic and chronic civilization complaints *without* the side effects of synthetic psycho pharmaceuticals.

A multicentered, double-blind study was conducted in 1974 to survey the effects of the KMG mixture on symptoms and conditions that were mostly results of autonomic nervous system imbalances (such as heart arrhythmia and similar heart conditions, dizziness, hot flashes, blushing, cold hands and feet, nervous perspiration, migraines, headaches). Significant improvement of the clinical state of all patients was found. A closer analysis showed primarily that the symptoms characteristic of vegetative disturbances (autonomic nervous system imbalances) had improved, mainly inner restlessness, unaccountable excitability, blushing, palpitation headaches, and other psychological indicators. The study showed a significant improvement in the area of ego strength as opposed to ego weakness according to standardized psychological profiles.[20] Highly significant improvements were found in the areas of nervousness and excitability. Treatments with a mixture of terpenoids as contained in Klosterfrau Melissengeist showed immense improvements in emotional stability. The results reliably supported use of these terpenoids for their positive therapeutic effect on all problems related to autonomic nervous system imbalances.

In another study of the same mixture, the treatment increased the ability to concentrate and improved depressive states.[21] Mental exhaustion, nervousness, and anxiety as well as physical disturbances such as heart pain, dizziness, headaches, lack of appetite, and gastrointestinal complaints improved dramatically.

Against viruses

A landmark study on the broad antiviral effects of essential oils and essential oil components was presented at the 1st Wholistic and Scientific Conference on the Therapeutic Uses of Essential Oils, 1995.[22] In this study, the broad spectrum of activity of essential oils and their components, as well as the effectiveness of those substances for conditions of the upper respiratory tract, skin, gastrointestinal tract, urogenital tract, nervousness, and arterial conditions was demonstrated. An overview of the antibacterial and antifungal effectiveness of essential oils and their components was given. Against many different species of bacteria, cinnamic aldehyde, cinnamic acid, eugenol, thymol, and black pepper oil were shown to be strongly effective. A strong antifungal effect was demonstrated for cinnamic aldehyde, black pepper oil, clove oil, eugenol, and thymol. Aflatoxin-forming fungi were shown to be inhibited by cinnamon oil, clove oil, and eugenol.[23] Recent in-vitro tests allow the quantitative proof of the antiviral effectiveness of different essential-oil constituents with specific consideration given to their cell toxic effects on human cells. Cinnamon oil, cinnamic aldehyde, black pepper oil, eugenol, and a range of terpenoids and phenylpropanoids show antiviral effects against herpes and adeno viruses with a rather broad spectrum of activity. The antiviral effectiveness of cinnamic aldehyde, black pepper oil, and the mix of KMG terpenes could be shown curatively as well as preventively in animal experiments after otherwise lethal herpes injections were administered. Cinnamic aldehydes and the terpenes of the KMG composition induce a significant increase of immunoglobulins.

That there are not more studies is a clear demonstration of the economic interests governing the scientific process. Given the extremely favorable track record of essential oils in treating viral diseases, one would expect researchers to jump on this opportunity to study cures that could be effective and, being relatively inexpensive, available to all. But again, since oils cannot be patented and scientists are economically dependent, these potential cures elicit mostly yawns from the scientific establishment. The advantages of aromatherapy remain outside of science. Those willing to try aromatherapy will find nontoxic and effective solutions for herpes simplex and herpes zoster simply with topical application of certain essential oils. As Schumacher commented years ago, "the direction of science cannot be left to the scientists."[24] Creating more complexity is easy. Seeing the simple and effective is next to impossible.

Wagner and Deininger postulated interaction between essential-oil components and receptors as early as 1973, but only lately have there been studies that actually corroborate these assumptions. Some of the most interesting results with respect to essential oils and receptor interaction shall be included here because they are excellent examples toward the beginning of a new understanding of many of the most outstanding health benefits of essential oils. Perhaps the most interesting recent study has come out of Sweden: "Terpenes Enhance Metabolic Activity and Alter Expression of Adhesion Molecules on Human Granulocytes."[25] This illustrates what aromatherapy asserted all along, that terpenes increase immune system and metabolic activity. To this end terpenes are able to change the expression of receptors, meaning that they are able to alter the amount of receptors present on the cell surface, either increasing or decreasing them.

Various metabolic cellular activities are associated with terpene exposure. These include induction of phase one and two hepatic detoxification enzymes, selective inhibition of protein isoprenylation, inhibition of coenzyme Q synthesis, and induction of receptors.[26] As a result, limonene and related terpenoids have been shown to prevent carcinogen-induced mammary cancer at both the initiation and the progression stages. Limonene causes complete regression of the majority of advanced rat mammary cancer when it is added to the diet. The interaction between sesquiterpenes and surface receptors has also been documented in different instances.

The probing of terpene, sesquiterpene, and receptor interaction has just begun. Throughout evolution, those substances with the most effective profile of interactions produce the greatest advantages for survival. A long-ranging and tedious selection has already happened over millions of years. These evolutionary selection processes cannot easily be replicated in the lab. There could be an endless number of such interactions, which may be researched only slowly, one by one. At this point, it can not be expected that interest in terpene action alone will generate any of that research. Some exceptions exist: the well-known sedative action of valerian root has led to studies on the interaction between the components of valerian and the GABA receptor in the brain, through which some of the known effects of valerian are presumed to be mediated.[27] In a study that has already triggered follow-up work, sesquiterpenes were shown to increase the number of certain receptors in the brain and are now considered prospects for the treatment of Alzheimer's, Parkinson's disease, and schizophrenia.[28] Close to the framework of aromatherapy, the interaction of sesquiterpenes from the essential oil of myrrh with various receptors were investigated.[29] Myrrh sesquiterpenes have similar or the same effects as opioid agonists, which explains the analgesic effect of the oil and its medical use in the past. Sesquiterpenes were found to be receptor stimulants, useful in the prevention and treatment of bronchial asthma, and components of vetiver oil inhibit the binding of vasopressin and, therefore, exert distinct influences on the tonus of the blood vessels.[30] Juvenile hormones, sesquiterpene derivatives, regulate reproductive developments.[31] In this case the receptor site is not situated on the surface but on the nucleus of the cell. Sesquiterpenes also are effective enhancers of penetration on human skin.[32]

Skin treated with the sesquiterpenes allows polar compounds such as water to penetrate more effectively.

The evolution of infectious disease in public consciousness

Over time, research follows trends. The discoveries of Pasteur and Koch and the emergence of the powerful concept of pathogenic microbes (germ-theory) influenced original research on the effects of essential oils. Antiseptic and antibacterial properties form the origin of our understanding of the pharmacology of essential oils, and it is worthwhile to reflect a moment on the path of these discoveries.

Recently, a surge in studies of sesquiterpene receptor interaction has occurred. Two factors are primarily responsible for this: among the complex molecular structures of sesquiterpenes, novel compounds can still be easily discovered, and two chemists and pharmacologists are inherently biased in favor of the effects of novel compounds, because they can be patented. Previously known effects of compounds are, comparatively, often neglected.

Following is a table of the trends of public awareness and the development of medical sciences.

Table 6.4: Events relating to aromatherapy and the public perception of science and medicine

1857	Pasteur	Fermentation caused by microorganisms; rabies vaccine
1876	Koch	Anthrax and the effect of turpentine on its spores; discovery of tuberculosis bacterium
1884	Wallach	Identification of the first terpenes; abandons sesquiterpene research
1910	Semmler	First correct structure of a sesquiterpene (ß-santalene)
1913	Kerschbaum	Discovery of precise molecular structure of farnesene

1920	Charabot & Dupont	Attempt first categorization of essential-oil constituents according to their chemical structure, mainly based on the functional groups encountered in aromatic molecules
1929	Fleming	Discovery of penicillin
1932	Domagk	Sulfanilamide
1937	Gattefossé	*Aromathérapie: Les Huiles essentielles, hormones végétales* summarizes known body of essential oil knowledge, coins the word "aromatherapy"
1939	Ruzicka	Nobel prize for elucidating the molecular structure of musk and other large-ring molecules
1943		First spraying of DDT for health reasons
1944	Dubos	First antibiotics production
1947	Robinson	Nobel prize for isoprene rule
1955	Salk	Polio vaccine
1955-59		Fifties optimism
1958-63		Malaria eradication efforts
1963	Rachel Carson	*The Silent Spring*
1964	Jean Valnet	*Aromathérapie* , which summarizes and reviews the work of earlier authors and creates a modernized system for the prescription of essential oils. In this period of emerging glory for antibiotics, Valnet is one of the isolated representatives of natural therapeutics. He founds the journal *Docteur Nature,* and the Association of Study and Research in Aromatherapy and Phytotherapy to which some of the foremost French representatives of aromatic medicine would belong. The publication of his book was an initial catalyst for broad popularization of aromatherapy.
1973	Pert	Discovery of the opiate receptor
1973	Wagner & Sprinkmeyer	Demonstration of sedative and spasmolytic effects of oils

1974	Deininger	Clinical proof, double-blind studies on effectiveness of essential oil for autonomic nervous system imbalances
1978	Belaiche	Publishes textbook on clinical application of aromatherapy
1980s	König	Enantioselective analysis and species specific isotope distribution
1981		First documented AIDS case
1983	Viaud	Emphasis on authentic essential oils for aromatherapy
1987	Deininger	Demonstrates antiviral properties of essential oils
1988	Origins	Estée Lauder becomes first large-scale corporation to use unadulterated essential oils in cosmetics
1990		Sesquiterpene receptor interaction becomes a research topic
1994	Preston	*The Hot Zone*; viruses become entertainment

"To teach doubt and experiment certainly was not what Christ meant."
—William Blake

SEVEN

A New Economy of Healing

Is aromatherapy up and coming?

Is aromatherapy going to be the "next big thing," a growing market with enormous potential?[1] There are no aromatherapy businesses becoming multimillion dollar businesses overnight. Those companies offering real aromatherapy in North America are small, often owner-operated. They are often small import companies that do not purchase essential oils from established fragrance brokers but import small quantities of essential oils from often similarly small distillers around the globe.[2] Other aromatherapy businesses are built around the therapeutic use of such genuine oils. Often there is emphasis on education, with the intent of empowering the layperson to responsibly use essential oils.

Financially, aromatherapy is not the most attractive option. High administrative costs—importation, custom clearance, small scale bottling, less than high-end packaging—are incurred by small businesses with limited sales. The logical conclusion is that the magic must be elsewhere. And indeed these enterprises are quite a new form of business. True aromatherapy enterprises really are different because for most operators the content—aromatherapy—

means more than the business. Aromatherapy is a business for those whose ideals and motivations are true.

In fact, those companies that have increased their sales into the multimillion-dollar range did so by leaving the concepts of vitalist aromatherapy behind, adjusting their products toward a gift- and cosmetic market with slickly packaged mass-market products of lesser meaning. An examination of current notions about medicine, essential oils, and money helps us understand where all of this might lead.

The pharmaceutical industry thrives on expensive drugs that millions of people take over long periods—years or decades—of time. Real money is involved. Aromatherapy does not offer such steep returns; is not *money medicine*. At first glance, the field of aromatherapy may seem to be wealthy, judging from the small vials filled with precious liquids. But this is an illusion based on the fact that we pay out-of-pocket money for oils and the expense is directly visible. Insurance holders rarely pay full price for their medicaments. The real costs of the treatments and services provided by conventional "money medicine" remain veiled by layers of administrative insulation while almost obscene premiums are raked in by health-insurance bureaucracies.[3] Some very slick strategies are at work. First, the public is constantly indoctrinated by the private sector to believe that government bureaucracies are costly and ineffective. Everyone is convinced that bureaucracy is exclusive to government and everything corporate is the height of efficiency. This is the disguise under which the health-insurance system, one of the most ineffective and hilariously expensive bureaucracies, can lead its parasitic life. The amount of money spent to administer the money spent on medicine is staggering. Meanwhile, alternative modalities such as aromatherapy perform just fine without creating such capitalistic bureaucracies.

A monopoly in a free-market economy

Examining the way pharmaceutical drugs are created is highly informative. The sums required for pharmaceutical research, clinical trials, and other procedures necessary for drug approval are to the tune of tens or hundreds of millions of dollars. Analyzing the details of this process for drugs approved in the recent past reveals bare-knuckle power plays by pharmaceutical giants in an attempt to get their new potential money-makers through this process.[4] Despite what the public is led to believe, scientific accountability routinely becomes an expendable nuisance, as studies are doctored and data is massaged to gain acceptance.[5] What emerges is a picture of unholy tinkering between regulators and corporate giants with all parties involved pretending to be motivated by goodness. That these industries get away with milking society for astronomical sums of money for what are at best dubious contributions seems quite Orwellian in its reversal of values. To ensure continuation of this scheme, a two-pronged strategy remains in place. It consists of: making sure that the majority of the population is absolutely convinced that the pharmaceutical industry has the interests of the people at heart, and insulating the existing system through legislation, thus giving the industry a monopoly in the medical field.

Once we are convinced that the ambitions of the pharmaceutical industry benefit our health, signs of the self-serving nature of this business are dismissed as an occasional excess or excusable lapses. The original intent, more drugs to improve human lives, is never doubted. As already discussed, the constant barrage of sensationalized reports on new medical breakthroughs cements the belief that a medical practice based on well-funded research will deliver new and better cures tomorrow. The mantra of progress hammers home the existing paradigm and makes it inappropriate to question it.

It is ironic that in the North American economic system, makers of medical drugs are allowed to operate under the protection of what amounts to a bona fide monopoly. The operating territories and thus profits for drug companies are protected by law. An obsolete interpretation of the scientific paradigm delivers the justification for this by branding everything that is not produced by the conventional process "quackery." The official position of recognizing only conventional drug therapy stubbornly reflects the state of thinking fifty years ago. How obsolete this way of thinking is is reflected by the fact that an age-old modality like acupuncture was also considered quackery by that part of the mainstream until recently.

Nonetheless, alternative methods grow in popularity. Hospitals, not directly involved in the manufacture of pharmaceuticals, are forced to recognize the trend. Recognizing the preferences of patients for alternative methods, some hospitals incorporate aromatherapy gadgetry to lure patients away from conservative institutions that do not offer these options. If these trends catch on, perhaps the rules to protect the monopoly will tighten in response. Ultimately, such measures will not stem the tide towards holistic health. New ways of thinking about the economic realities of the conventional medical system have emerged recently. The staggering cost of the conventional system is seen not only as an almost unbearable burden but also as a gigantic opportunity.

A statement by Schumacher describes the predicament of the conventional system aptly: "The most striking thing about modern industry is that it requires so much and accomplishes so little. Modern industry seems to be inefficient to a degree that surpasses one's ordinary powers of imagination. Its inefficiency therefore remains unnoticed." This is only too true for the medical industry. The amounts of money spent in the pressing areas of cancer, upper respiratory diseases, and intestinal diseases are ludicrous. It is only a matter of time until more competitive offerings will provide better solutions for less money. Michio Kaku, in *Visions* seems to agree: "The problem is that the drug companies have to spend a large amount of resources on new medicines. Because it often takes ten to fifteen years and $300 million to bring a new drug onto the market, we may be defenseless against certain resistant diseases early in the next century."[6]

Kaku's statement is highly indicative of the factors at play, the first of which is the acceptance and reliance of technical developments with no questioning of the social and political parameters influencing them. Drugs supposedly *have* to be that expensive. Actually, it is possible to manufacture and offer products that require equal amounts of research for minimal amounts of money (such as appetite suppressants and other over-the-counter drugs) when there is no insurance institution behind the potential customer and the manufacturer has to rely on the ability of the end-consumer to afford the product. The next factor at play is the accepting as inevitable that resistant diseases developed as a consequence of man's attempts to play God.

In the long run, the ethics of a society determine its economic order. In Western societies, especially in North America, economics are structured in very close alignment with the prevailing individualistic ethic. Economic actions and structure are, therefore, an expression of individual desires—whether a single person, a group, or a company—for personal gain or career advancement. Individualistic, entrepreneurial effort shapes the innovative processes in this society. The same individualistic principle shapes the innovative process within the medical industrial complex. This is probably not the most promising concept toward furthering public and individual health.

The causes of misery and disease

In a society totally devoted to free-market economy, the well-being of one and the misery of others is attributed to an individual's skill, willingness to work and take risks, and entrepreneurial spirit. According to free-market ideology, the best solutions or products supposedly will arise through natural selection. But the process is brutal.

In the United States, where market economics is practiced most uninhibitedly, the consequence are obvious. Society is not only distinguished by high mobility, flexibility, freedom, and an abundance of ideas and innovative concepts, but also by a high degree of inequality, hyper-materialism, crime, violence, a constant rise of psychological disorders, and a drug subculture out of control (all this can be summarized as representing the entropic sector of society). Is there a more humane and intelligent way to provide the benefits of a working-market mechanism than this brutal spectacle?

A contribution in the winter 1996 issue of *Taipan*, a newsletter alerting investors to market trends before they become common knowledge, makes some interesting points. It shows that a growing revolt against the United States' medical establishment is exhibited not only by supporters of alternative medicine but also by conservative minds.

Use of all types of alternative medicine is on the increase with billions of dollars at stake. *The New England Journal of Medicine* notes that one-third of all doctor's visits are to non-M.D.s. *Taipan* observes that a breed of "new aristocrats" are leading the way in this revolt. It seems that the high-income and higher-education demographic profiles also show a high incidence of turning to alternative solutions for back pain, heart disease, cancer, allergies, multiple sclerosis—virtually all diseases for which the medical establishment has no answers. If you are an American with cancer, some would say the smartest thing to do would be to get on a plane and leave the country as many of the most progressive cancer treatments are unavailable, not to mention illegal, here. To medical doctors, the body is a machine. You cut it open, fix it, replace parts. But more and more of us are not buying into body mechanics. We can live up to a hundred years—in fact the natural limit to our life span is roughly 120. Living healthily is the key, not getting a doctor to fix you once you have broken down. *Taipan* predicts more and more people are going to take their health into their own hands, resulting in new industries.[7]

The same basic direction can also be encountered in a current economic theory that argues that the cost associated with the entropic sector of society will become the motor for future economic development.[8] While information-processing in any form is still the biggest sector of the global economy, *content* is not a priority. This lack of content is one of the main reasons for the high cost of the entropic aspects of society. A movement toward content will gain increasing importance for many forms of alternative healing, and methods with a more integrative attitude toward health and humans will tap this huge entropic reservoir.

In economic terms, these are enormous energy reserves that can

Table 7.1: Economic impact of the side effects of techno-civilization

Crime and drugs

- Cost of burglary, theft, murder, bodily injury, and so on worldwide costs more than a thousand billion dollars per year. Every fiftieth American was in prison in the mid 1990s.
- Illegal drugs cost more than eight hundred billion dollars per year.
- Bribery and corruption make up 3 to 5 percent of the cost of all economic activity (worldwide about a thousand billion dollars).
- Alcohol: more than six hundred billion dollars spent per year (more money is spent on alcohol than on research).
- Every fourth fire of industrial installations in the million-dollar range is a result of arson.

Environmental destruction, unemployment

- Annual destruction of the environment is equivalent to about 10 percent of the gross global product (GGP), more than $2,700 billion annually.
- Eighty percent of all finished products are discarded after the first use. Resulting annual waste of energy (worldwide) is a minimum of twenty-five hundred billion dollars.
- Cost of unemployment is more than three hundred billion dollars per year in industrial nations.

Other damages and costs

- Psychological dysfunctions: Fourteen percent of the population in economically developed countries suffer from serious psychological illnesses. Sixty percent of Germans in leading positions are considered neurotic, and 30 percent of German employees occasionally feel like strangling their bosses. In Germany, mobbing causes annual damages of thirty billion dollars; two hundred billion dollars worldwide.
- Deterioration of families: One half of all marriages in the United States end in divorce.

- Poor technology: Office workers have to spend 20 percent of their working time repairing malfunctioning computers or programs.
- Patents: Fifty percent of all research and development expenses are redundant and could be saved (almost three hundred billion dollars in the United States.)
- Cost caused by traffic jams is over a thousand billion dollars worldwide.
- There are counterproductive developments in health care, such as a rise in misdiagnosis, malpractice, and mistakes due to lack of knowledge. Nutritional mistakes alone incur six hundred billion dollars in health costs worldwide.

be used for improvement and increased productivity of society at large. Reversing only a small fraction of the psycho-social ills represents big economic gains. The losses modern society suffers through psychological disorders, violence, crime, drugs, environmental destruction, and other damaging factors represent a staggering ten thousand billion dollars. A third of the world's GGP is lost through these misguided energies, and as the past has amply demonstrated, these factors are not reversed by more sophisticated technological innovations. Instead, they put more demands on the physical, mental, and psychological (emotional) resources of individuals. Through the disintegration of family, private life is becoming less of a place to turn to for quietude and regeneration. Quiet, connection to nature, holistic health and happiness, and many other contributing factors to well-being are in short supply. Alternative methods such as aromatherapy offer great potential where physical healing and psychological regeneration intersect, because they provide integrated solutions. So far this potential has been suffocated by restrictive legislation.

This correlation may be clearly noted in the rise of psychological problems and disease. In the United States, where treatment of chronic depression alone costs forty-three billion dollars annually, 14 percent of the population is considered to be seriously psychologically ill. The economic aspects of these problems are often not realized to their full extent.

A socially tolerable deregulation of the health-care market will unleash enormous economic development. A sensible approach to

Table 7.2: Annual cost of diseases in the United States

Cancer	$104 billion
Lethal respiratory	$99 billion
AIDS	$66 billion
Lethal heart disease	$32 billion
Arthritis	$38 billion
Schizophrenia	$33 billion

alternative healing does not mean the encouragement of profiteering quackery. The shift of demand from material goods to demand for social, emotional, and physical well-being will be the strongest economic trend of the foreseeable future. This will be the first time where economic development is not dependent on raw materials, hardware, or computers but on progress in the area of human life. The true innovation will lie in the development of psycho-social potentials or, as a headline in *UTNE Reader* refered to it, "the most important development in the near future might not be a new technology but human spirit."

Diseases of the mind and soul

Alternative modalities such as aromatherapy offer useful strategies for dealing with current civilization diseases. Conditions such as cancer, AIDS, heart disease, and arthritis correspond to alienation brought on by industrial lifestyles. The notion of separation of body, mind, and soul is fruitless, because whether we like it or not our body is a web of interacting systems. This gap between the old systems and the proposals for an integrative approach to healing represents the biggest economic possibilities of the future. The potential is most obvious with solutions for allergies, autonomic nervous-system dysfunctions, and psychological problems such as addiction to drugs or prescription pharmaceuticals. While the old medical system clings to its outdated dogma, the possibilities for holistic healing are huge: in industrialized countries approximately one sixth of the GNP is spent on health care (a thousand billion dollars in the United States) and this volume is rising rapidly, pointing to the dynamic nature of this industry. If other industries benefiting health are included, such as food, ecological conservation, sports, or certain aspects of tourism, the total volume allocated to health care rises to one fourth of the GNP.

Historical considerations point to health as the new major economy. Industrialization, which had been the motor of economic development since the eighteenth century, has passed its peak with the dawn of the information age. Industry will retain some importance—the supply of goods of all kinds from manufacturing industries will continue and will remain a major factor—but it has lost its ability to usher in new trends, as less than 20 percent of all employees work in the manufacturing industry.

Industrialization created an enormous abundance of goods, but it also created most of the psychological and physical health problems discussed in this book. With material goods readily available and the information technology unable to fill the void of content, the desire for physical and psychological health will be the biggest demand of the future. Only alternative, holistic modalities lead to an improved command of the phenomena of the soul, which is necessary to satisfy these needs.

"...immense technological development causes gridlocks and malfunctions. The vastly expanded alimentary industry has converted to the production of poisonous and carcinogenic foods."
—Umberto Eco, *Travels in Hyperreality*

EIGHT

Healing and Belief

Essential oils were once held in high regard, and based on an improved understanding of their almost limitless complexity and biological compatibility, there is every reason to believe that this will happen again. As a true healing modality, aromatherapy straddles two paradigms, the old scientific/mechanistic view of medicine and an emerging new paradigm that recognizes the reality of the physical body but also respects those of the mind and the soul. The importance of consciousness is illustrated by a story at the beginning of *Beyond Antibiotics*, by Michael A. Schmidt, Lendon H. Smith, and Keith W. Sehnert.[1]

In March 1991, I appeared on a Miami radio program with two holistic physicians. The topic was how we manage and prevent infections using nutrition, botanical medicine and other means. The discussion eventually centered on the health of our own children. One doctor commented that of his five children between the ages of three and thirteen, none had ever received antibiotics. I added that my then three-week-old son had also never been on antibiotics. Several weeks later, I spoke with a nurse who was the wife of a holistic physician. Of their nine children between the ages of three and twenty-one, none had ever been treated with antibiotics.

This was astonishing. Was it possible that these children never got sick? Had they never suffered from bacterial (or viral) infections? What was the magic formula that allowed all these families to avoid antibiotic use while their friends and neighbors received the drugs for many common ailments? While generally very healthy, these children did experience bacterial and viral infections like all other children (although less frequent). However, rather than being treated with antibiotics, which kill germs, but do nothing else for the child, they were treated with immune-building alternatives. The course of their illnesses were generally very short and recurrent infections were rare.

This was in stark contrast to the families of a group of family practice residents I was recently asked to speak to at a large Minneapolis hospital. The problem: their own children were constantly sick and were on antibiotics off-and-on for the better part of the winter. The children were sickly, coughing and had perpetual runny noses. These physicians wondered if there was any way they could improve the health of their children and get them off antibiotics. (The view changes when it hits close to home!) They were frustrated by the limitations of using antibiotics alone and hoped I might provide them with information on using diet, nutrition, herbs, acupressure, and other ways of boosting immunity.

The differences between the families just described reflect a basic difference in philosophy. The holistic doctor views the patient as a whole and directs treatment to the patient during infection. The allopathic doctor typically views this type of illness as the result of bacterial invasion. Their treatment is directed toward the bacteria. We are of the former philosophy. We believe there are better ways to approach illness than the means being used by most allopathic doctors today.

This story is a perfect example of the enormous influence the mind can have on physical health.

The conditioning rendered by soft-spoken, glossy, double-page ads of caring pharmaceutical companies and the never-ending news of the medical breakthrough of the day make their mark. But true healing—strengthening the fabric of life—does not usually come in a pill box. It takes conscious effort not to allow one's perceptions to be shaped by forces from outside.

The most difficult step is to give up the belief that the old system is somehow always a little bit more right than the new. Most everyone in contemporary Western societies was raised to do as the doctor ordered and to accept any outcome as the best possible solution. The medical industry does everything in its power to maintain this image of benevolent authority.

One tactic is to brand the desire for natural treatments as irresponsible behavior. Often, doctors or nurses make people who want to utilize natural ways of healing feel like unruly children, not behaving as authority has prescribed. Many patients have been convinced that they may not take responsibility for their own health. As a result, the *pretense* of responsibility falls to the medical system with consequences that are rarely scrutinized. One only need examine the whole set of assumptions that lie behind the accepted fact that doctors decide who can stay home from work.

One of the most effective means of manipulating the public to firmly believe in the status quo is to imply authority indirectly. This is reflected in the question of whether or not aromatherapy is "recognized." Recognized by whom? Tacitly implied is an understanding that any new modality must be approved by the holy bureau of the old paradigm. All this does is insure continued suppression of alternate methods. A feature article in a German weekly, investigating alternative health modalities, illustrates this. Conventional physicians were asked to evaluate the modalities. The verdict for most was a condescending "probably harmless but also useless." Compliance with the old paradigm is solicited with the lament that the danger lies in keeping unsuspecting patients away from superior and truly effective conventional treatments. No, aromatherapy is not recognized but this is good news.

Specialized care and the denial of dignity

What has specialized, technologically and pharmaceutically driven medicine done for us? It has made any occurrence of even the most common condition such as the flu a depressing and difficult episode, and, through its relentless overmedication, added to the problem by creating more chronic illness. It has robbed our experience of being ill of all the empowering aspects that can be found in the process and replaced them with rigid protocols.

Becoming ill used to be a fact of life and included such human aspects as being cared for by a grandmother, having extra time to read, and so on. The entire process, within the whole fabric of an individual's life, has its rightful place. Often, bodies simply require downtime. Now being ill means having one's symptoms managed with mass-market products. Worse is the demeaning way in which the manufacturer assumes that the prospective customers are dumb enough to make grossly inadequate use of the medication; medicine pamphlets are now worded to insulate the maker from liability.

The exclusively for-profit nature of the system does not even allow time for the most intimate human moments and experiences. Are extremely expensive chemotherapy products sold out of concern for patients or to cash in on in extreme despair? Whatever the answer might be, the issues of the dignity of a dying human being and the potential to make one final big sale are terribly mixed up. Finding out how pharmaceutical giants in the late seventies and early eighties predicted the rise in cancer and carefully plotted their vastly increased future income through extremely expensive chemotherapy does not help to restore our trust in the money medicine.[2]

Medical products are sold not unlike cars or vacuum cleaners in that they are not designed for individuals but for the masses. Mass medicine is inherently infested with dangerous and even fatal side-effects and is inherently damaging to a large number of people. Even if a medicine drug "works," it produces side-effects—often clearly admitted in the studies performed for approval of the drug. The argument is that a certain amount of risk is acceptable if a larger percentage will benefit. But whose logic is that? The logic of the risk group or the vendor? Personal health is difficult or impossible to calculate by anonymous statistics.

We need not regress to past methods, but we must understand the conditions of the present. The challenge is not to throw out scientific evidence that was gained but to overcome the soulless hyper-materialism that came with it. Materialism pertaining to the manufacture of consumer goods and clever exploitation of the earth's resources seemed tolerable simply because it was far enough away to be blissfully ignored. But as the same ideologies hit the bodies in which we live, we are forced to think harder.

Medical hexing

Sometimes the medical system becomes so self-absorbed in its authority that gross abuses are accepted as scientific accuracy, particularly with regard to physicians (usually specialists) making predictions on the outcome of a disease or guessing how much time a patient has left to live. Andrew Weil calls this "medical hexing." Such guesswork either develops into self-fulfilling prophecies or requires the almost superhuman energies of a patient to overcome it. Wasn't it the obligation of the physician in the first place to help the patient overcome the condition? Medical hexing, the overvaluing of intervention, and the belief in specialization all work together to undermine an individual's resolve to become active in the process. How does this happen? Certainly doctors making such statements do not act out of bad intentions; to the contrary the physician most likely acts under the impression that it is her or his duty to inform a patient fully.

Taking control

Modalities such as aromatherapy present corrective challenges to the destructive dynamics of one-dimensional progress, which is aptly defined as "better living through technology." The challenge comes from a renewed appreciation of the phenomenon of life in general. All of a sudden, women have begun to explore healing with the use of plants, the way it was done long before science ever came around. Especially in high-tech societies, essential oils present a growing attraction.

There are rumblings of a new appreciation of the forces of life. The wildly exaggerated projections of the mechanistic worldview are questioned from many different vantage points by contemporary writers. The dusty, mechanistic notion of the body is crumbling in its wake. The one-dimensional cause-and-effect models that modern medicine has exploited so effectively are no longer fit to describe reality even for those who choose to align their worldview to the trends of science. As the new discoveries invalidate science's old dogmas, new forms of submission are introduced. The connection between emotional well-being and immune status were known to people long before there was scientific proof. The arrogance of the old paradigm is expressed in belief that something cannot be taken as real unless it is scientifically proven. Only after science corroborates an age-old traditional treatment may the imbecile public accept it as reality and use it. It is the most blatant admission of hubris, that scientific proof amounts to the act of creation.

The admission that self-healing occurs is another challenge to the mechanistic model and economic projection of medicine, and reveals the very wise reactions of the body in crisis. The self-healing abilities of the body have been there all along but are now being brilliantly rediscovered in books such as Andrew Weil's *Spontaneous Healing*. Because alternative therapies often force radical changes in thinking—leading to the recognition of the emotional, moral, and spiritual void at the root of civilization diseases—they are more effective in treating them. Aromatherapy allows space to be intuitive and to reconnect with nature, because it is not possible to solve the crisis with the means that created it in the first place. The modern view of man on top of nature is obsolete. Living healthily and happily requires unison with the world around us.

The issue at hand is how to relate to science, which in many aspects has provided the basis of existence in Western societies despite instincts and rational thinking that favor more holistic healing modalities. The conditioning is only gradually removed from our minds. The answer is to utilize what science has given us but also to unlock the many powers to heal that are beyond the command of conventional medicine.

In Greek mythology, there are two opposing views: doctors who believe in outside intervention to cure disease (conventional approach) and healers (often laypeople) who believe in maintaining health through following the natural order of things (holistic approach). These two views were personified by Asklepios, the god of medicine (conventional system), and Hygieia, his daughter, goddess of health.

Our total reliance on chemical and surgical intervention and weaponry to kill germs is the modern manifestation of the Asklepian approach. It neglects the importance of keeping a body in balance. Sooner or later, relying on weaponry creates casualties. Today many conventional drugs are known to weaken immune response and lead to a wide range of undesirable effects. That drugs sometimes bring on exactly those diseases that they are meant to cure is a bitter reality.

Conversely, the Hygieian approach focuses on strengthening health and building resistance. Given the choice, wouldn't everyone rather strengthen the body's own defense system and enjoy health rather than allow disease to appear only to treat it later (the conventional approach). In theory, yes. But the promises of modern medicine have blinded many into accepting its hubris as a sustainable reality. Often it is difficult to recognize the fallacies and to leave the perceived haven of modern medicine for modalities that subject us to uncomfortable admissions: we are mortal and we need to cooperate with nature instead of trying to master it. After negative experiences that reveal the hubris of techno-medicine we learn to appreciate the softer methods.

After contrasting the *claims* of the pharmacological system with reality, the conclusion can only be that while medicine has brought valuable contributions to human welfare, its purported infallibility is a hoax. Nonetheless, decades of conditioning will not just go away; it has become part of our makeup. Sometimes there are no perfect solutions, and doing the little that can be done is still a forceful way to outgrow the disenchantment wrought by the old system. What is required is curiosity and a softening of one's convictions. Aromatherapy can help. Renewal happens in more ways than expected when lavender is applied to a burn and, surprisingly, the next morning the skin is intact and the pain is gone. Shifts in thinking can also occur through the use of essential oils in winter, as people learn how to manage bronchitis or a case of the flu by keeping symptoms at a minimum and coming out of it stronger than before. (See page 230.) These experiences create powerful changes. Management of these conditions with natural means strengthens the immune system, and previously frequent conditions reappear less or disappear completely. This leads to taking more responsibility for the health of family members. Aromatherapy starts this dynamic process through its immediate connection with mind and emotion. The safest way to successful self-care and reclaimed responsibility consists of moderate yet deliberate steps. Initial possibilities include using relaxing and pleasantly soothing oils such as lavender or clary sage for de-stressing baths or massages. A great "entry-level" essential oil for natural medicine is tea tree oil *(Melaleuca alternifolia)*, which is nontoxic and proven effective for the treatment of nonspecific bladder infections. Similarly, there are a number of essential oils that provide effective relief for herpes simplex lesions. Once set in motion, a new appreciation of the power of natural healing will continue to grow.

Allowing simplicity

The potential hazards of essential-oil use are limited and easy to keep in mind (some of the hazards are listed in the table on page 174). These hazards should be seen as only moderate dangers—with only a minimum of common sense, the hazards can easily be avoided. Again, most of these substances have a millions-of-years-old history of interaction with other organisms. The aromatherapy enthusiast does not need to worry about a surprise occurrence of toxic materials in his or her essential oils—as long as the oils are genuine and authentic. This is in stark contrast to conventional drugs, which usually have noticeable side effects and *seem* safe but nonetheless lead to the deaths of roughly a hundred thousand people annually.

One of the most puzzling problems for any newcomer—and even for advanced aromatherapy enthusiasts—is the broad interchangeability of oils that is often possible (without loss of effectiveness). Very often conditions respond to the use of essential oils regardless of which oils are being used. It appears to be the implementation of aromatherapy alone which brings improvement. This is patently unsettling to our scientifically conditioned minds. In spite of the fact that oils have distinct pharmacological properties, healing is often achieved just by using an oil, no matter which one. Remembering that terpenes increase metabolic activity is a good way to begin to understand this.

One example is the civilization disease neuro dermatitis. There are no known oils that would quickly and effectively cure this condition which, at least in a holistic view, is brought on by many of the factors present in today's urban lifestyle. When a condition is the expression of years of subscribing to a certain lifestyle, it is unlikely to be reversed instantaneously through the use of an essential oil. However, if an individual applies German chamomile to counteract the itching, a degree of symptomatic relief will take place. When complemented with lavender to relieve stress and rosemary and tarragon to recondition the gastrointestinal tract, increased metabolic activity will lead to elimination of toxins and re-equilibration of the nervous system. An overall improvement will occur and very likely contribute to a recovery from the condition. The results of such a treatment are not limited to the immediate effect of the applied oils, but include a cascade of developments following the first successful use. This cascade creates a gradual change in how the mind relates to aromatherapy. It serves to encourage a more natural lifestyle, the intake of fewer toxins, and so on—all factors that will ultimately benefit the recovery from complex civilization diseases.

The broad spectrum of effects makes a simple answer to the magic bullet or one-shot formula question (the routine question asked in aromatherapy seminars) so difficult. Because we're conditioned to have one specific substance for one specific condition, it is difficult to fathom that all these effects are stimulated by an oil or even three or four oils. No oil will cure a complex civilization condition, but using aromatherapy *will* still be beneficial. Aromatherapy favors the free flow of the communication molecules as well as a limbic and nervous system in balance. The need for allopathic drugs vanishes, ideally paving the way for a more balanced life.

Another mental obstacle presented by mechanistic conditioning is that we are bothered by not knowing which of a set of measures caused the improvement. But if healing occurs, does it matter which was the active step? It only matters if there is a commercial desire to bottle it and sell it. The truth is, there may not be one active element but a *combination* of activities that do the trick, including the fact that we get in the habit of taking better care of ourselves when we do more than just pop a pill. The resolve to take care of oneself can contribute greatly.

What should you do when bronchitis is coming on with a slight soreness in the throat and the early signs of a cold? A combination of supporting measures will help: upper chest rubs and inhalations with essential oils, sauna, Chinese herbs and/or propolis, and going to bed early. If, as a result of one or more of these measures, the bronchitis is warded off, that is the result. The question of which of the actual components of the treatment were the effective ones is secondary.

What about all that research?

Translating the scientific data on oils into therapeutic practice remains difficult because the expected step of applying research to establish treatment regimens, dosages, and marketable products is absent. This is one more challenge to the way we are conditioned to think. There really are no practicing aromatherapy experts in the sense that there are expert physicians. The majority of professionals who provide aromatherapy integrate it with whatever their profession is. This might seem a disadvantage at first, but it is not; in order to benefit from aromatherapy, one is forced to do it oneself. It is an active form of healing, not a conventional passive one. As a layperson, one is forced to either accept the available data as corroboration that the practices of aromatherapy make sense, or you simply go by intuition, books, or other forms of learning. Research results can be quite stimulating since they often explain scientifically what has been observed empirically. They provide support for exploring the best ways oils can be put to use. On the shaky ground between the paradigms, it turns out that healing is not the exclusive privilege of science. Aromatherapy reminds us that science needs to be complemented with respect for the immaterial phenomena of life.

In this respect aromatherapy is the future of healing. Essential oils, representatives of the plant world, communicate with all planes of human consciousness. This is a privilege of plant intelligence over synthetic drugs and the exclusive fixation on the corresponding material plane. Science is gradually learning how forces long thought irrelevant to therapeutic practice are in fact highly relevant. From prayer to hugs, from emotional influences on the immune status to the meaning of social ties and religious beliefs, science is waking up to the mind/body connection. But given the proven rigidity of the scientific process, it may well be too late when science will finally be able to integrate these concepts into treatments that its establishment approves of.

With or without science, essential oils are working. Aromatherapy is a contemporary reemergence of human and plant cooperation the way it used to be. Humans respond to oils because plants and people have always communicated in their own way.

"Auf die Stimme unserer Seele hören sollen, wenn wir gesunden wollen."
(If we want to heal, we should listen to the voices of our souls.)
—Hildegard von Bingen

NINE
Aromatherapy Delivers the Goods

Daniel Pénoël has called aromatic matter the immune system of humanity. This statement poetically points to the broad range of interaction possible between essential oils and humans. In this chapter some of the qualities shall be discussed that are specific to aromatherapy and at the core of its fascination.

Quasi medicine

For most newcomers to aromatherapy, its quasi medicinal aspects are accepted most easily and are therefore a common point of entry. In this mode, aromatherapy alleviates symptoms, basically mimicking the symptom-management principles of conventional medicine. This will indeed work and in the right cases even work very successfully. The casual user will be rewarded with some very real successes. The impact of the natural fragrances on the emotion-processing systems of brain and body may even initiate unexpected shifts of consciousness.[1]

Renewal

With aromatherapy, the sense of exploring true healing, the way Jane Achtenberg has defined it as strengthening the fabric of life, can be initiated. True healing happens when we are empowered to change those factors in life that are at the root of disease. It happens when we break the cycle of medication, doctor, and disease, and gradually enter a state of health. I would like to refer to this process as *renewal*. The great power of aromatherapy lies in its ability to precipitate this renewal, to set it in motion. We must, however, fully realize that, with the multitude and depth of health problems that can be encountered, trying to remedy every condition with aromatherapy alone would be futile. Aromatherapy, properly understood, will also lead the user to employ other modalities when appropriate.

Compared to other alternative methods, aromatherapy is uniquely safe and easy to use. It is advisable to take precautions (see page XX) but there is no need to imitate the intimidating procedures of conventional medicine.

Aromatherapy works by another standard—reasonable play. This is expressed in the way people fall in love with aromatherapy. A relationship develops quite similar to that of a couple falling in love. There is infatuation and the building of a useful and lasting partnership. The analogy goes even further: just as couples, throughout a long and successful partnership, develop more individual identity and sometimes divergent interests, similarly, acceptance of aromatherapy does not require the exclusion of other alternative methods but rather implores us to build a network of resources for maintaining a healthy balance and a lifestyle of renewal.

Manipulation versus self-correction

The inability of technology to recognize limitations has been described aptly by E. F. Schumacher:

> If that which has been shaped by technology, and continues to be so

> shaped, looks sick, it might be wise to have a look at technology itself. If technology is felt to be becoming more and more inhuman, we might do well to consider whether it is possible to have something better—a technology with a human face. Strange to say, technology, although of course the product of man, tends to develop by its own laws and principles, and these are very different from those of human nature or living nature in general. Nature always, so to speak, knows when and where to stop. Greater even than the mystery of natural growth is the mystery of the natural cessation of growth. There is measure in all natural things—in their size, speed, or violence. As a result, the system of nature, of which man is part, tends to be self-balancing, self-adjusting, self-cleansing. Not so with technology, or perhaps I should say: Not so with man dominated by technology and specialization. Technology recognizes no self-limiting principle—in terms, for instance, of size, speed, or violence. It therefore does not possess the virtues of being self-balancing, self-adjusting, and self-cleansing. In the subtle system of nature, technology, and in particular the super-technology of the modern world, acts like a foreign body, and there are now numerous signs of rejection (E. F. Schumacher).

Unlike manipulative modalities that are based on technology, aromatherapy is self-correcting. If errors are made in aromatherapy, they may be resolved through the discontinuation of the wrongful application of an oil. If an inflammation arises following the use of an irritant oil, it will dissipate as soon as the oil is discontinued *without* having caused any lasting damage. Aromatherapy makes it possible for the layperson to build a repertoire of experience from which to operate. The occasional mistake is never injurious, but instead provides valuable guidance how to correctly use the often underestimated power of essential oils. Because essential oils provide a generous margin for error, there is ample room to learn through inconsequential discomfort. With commercial drugs this is not the case, since they compete under conditions that make it necessary to pretend only pleasurable experiences can happen. Drugs are formulated to fit the market in a consumer society, not the needs of a person.

Two advantages of essential-oil therapy are the immediacy of its action and its tolerability and safety. There are many instructional books on aromatherapy that teach how to use essential oils in practical ways at home. But while many of these books mention the need for professional oversight or guidance, very few doctors could prescribe, much less know about, aromatherapy—especially in North America. Realistically, using essential oils is only possible in a self-medicating manner. R. Deininger, one of the most respected essential-oil researchers, concurs: "The main area for the use of the anti-microbial action of essential oils are trivial infections in the context of self-medication: Infections of the respiratory system (in combination with a spasmolytic action of essential oils), skin infections (e. g. herpes virus), diseases of the gastrointestinal tract (in combination with spasmolytic action), urinary tract infections (in connection with diuretic action). Advantages: broad spectrum of activity. Side-effects are not to be expected when the products are used properly."[2]

Is it safe?

While not impossible, it is extremely unlikely that a person would cause real injury through the use of essential oils. Compared to the serious problems of conventional medical practices and the havoc that drugs can cause, the potential for problems with aromatherapy is marginal to nonexistent. On the other hand, the likelihood of deriving great health benefits from oils (by reducing or completely eliminating antibiotics) is enormous. The instances of severe or fatal poisoning with plants are few, compared to those of conventional drugs.[3]

A reasonable discussion of the safety of essential oils is distorted by the demand for "absolute safety" by the consumer. These demands are usually entertained by commercial interest looking for a way to sell to a public perceived as underinformed. The real intent of these demands is to ensure safety for the business venture. Alarmist attempts to completely discontinue the use of certain oils are a result of this. These warnings are made because there is a fear that accidents with essential oils could be used by government organizations to prohibit trade and thus hurt business. In light of the potential benefits, a modality as safe as aromatherapy should continue to be accessible despite the fact that minor accidents may occur, especially because the probability is much lower than for any other form of self-medication.

Pregnancy

A large number of women in their child-bearing years are attracted to aromatherapy and the instinct to protect a growing baby is undeniable. Any evaluation of the safety of essential oils must begin with the consideration of possible alternatives. Say a pregnant woman contracts bronchitis of the lower respiratory tract. Should she choose the appropriate use of oregano oils, despite the fact that some books recommend against it, or should she turn to traditional medicine for her condition with a round of hard-hitting, immune-suppressing, and otherwise unpredictable antibiotics? Is it safer to expose the fetus to these modern drugs or to substances that have been around for millions of years? Not much is known about the safety of essential-oil use during pregnancy. Sweeping disclaimers are constantly established, banishing every essential oil that exhibits only a hint of a problem potential from use during pregnancy. But these highly defensive statements mostly ignore the potential for problems from the conventional drug alternatives. Obviously, disclaimers really are set up to protect the vendor and are of little help for women trying to decide between aromatherapy and drug therapy. The reasonable approach is to proceed with common sense and reason, to try and maintain balance and prevent infections during pregnancy with those essences that are known to be easy on the system, which we will later classify as "tonics of life." But, if specific or more severe conditions necessitated, one could arrive at the conclusion that even some of the more forceful use of essential oils might still be a much more reasonable approach than allopathic drugging. This is an area where communication between women would definitely provide more assurance and safety than arcane long-term research projects.

Returning healing power to women

The warlike fighting of disease is an expression of masculinity; *creatively* solving the problems of life is feminine.The violent tendencies of the scientific revolution are revealed in newspaper articles that describe medicine and medicinal research with the terminology of war: "developing new weapons against," "killing germs," "the cancer war," and so on. The language is male and defines our experience of medicine today.

That male ideology and parlance has been adopted as representative for both genders in the medical field may be at the core of the failures of conventional medicine. A painful awareness of losing battles in the "wars" against malaria, tuberculosis, cancer, and other diseases takes hold. Wars were waged by pouring DDT into tropical swamps, which proved toxic but ineffective: malaria and tuberculosis are coming back with a vengeance.[4] All these chemicals and drugs are like weapons. They are dangerous and need to be used with great care and discrimination to prevent them inflicting more harm than they already have. The hollowness becomes obvious when supposedly sacrosanct bulwarks of scientific objectivity and truth like the *New England Journal of Medicine* repeatedly need to engage in deceptive tactics such as allowing industrial apologists (chemicals salesmen) to pose as independent scientists to write editorials without revealing their commercial affiliations and interests.[5]

Could a more cooperative approach toward overcoming disease work better? In holistic modalities like aromatherapy (or TCM), well-rounded, complex mixtures of natural substances are used. Essential oils allow a woman to implement more of the Hygieian principle of strengthening and nurturing. Essential oils are also infinitely more pleasing aesthetically than chemical weaponry.

That the female approach works has been proven in the field of child-rearing. An undetermined but large percentage of mothers do their best to treat their children at home, *without* the use of antibiotics. This goes on despite exposure to the conventional system's conditioning and pressure tactics. Why do women search for alternatives? Why is maternal apprehension to administering allopathic medication on the rise?

Considering the devastating consequences of antibiotics use, we observe instinct outsmarting science; obviously, intuition led mothers to better judgment. Women who keep their children off of antibiotics have taken better care of their children's overall health than those who chose to medicate. (See page 114.) If the urge to keep children off allopathic medications stems from intuitive impulse, those instinctual and intuitive parts of our brain are ensuring survival even better than our highly touted rational abilities.

The purported inclusion of women into medicine is deceiving. True, medicine has opened up career opportunities for women, but only at the price of swallowing the basically male ideology of the system. With more space allotted for intuition, women find far more acceptance in alternative healing methods.

But even alternative modalities such as acupuncture require a high degree of expertise. Aromatherapy, however, is safe and effective for everyone, not just experts. This makes it easier for women to take care of the health of their family. One could even consider aromatherapy to be the primary health-care system of Western societies. Aromatherapy is a female modality that emphasizes female qualities and cooperative approaches. Because it is straightforward and effective in its application, it returns the power of healing back to the individual, especially to the individual woman. Aromatherapy liberates women from male medical pressure by providing effective alternatives.

As aromatherapy moves forward it will become increasingly more difficult to obscure its female nature and reality. There are encouraging signs that aromatherapy does indeed equip women to offer more cooperative healing than does the old paradigm. Because the effects of aromatherapy were too soft—they did not hit hard enough for corporate exploitation—it has been spared from becoming the object of male corporate hierarchies. It thrives in small businesses operated by women, many of whom imbue aromatherapy with idealistic ideas that venture beyond mere commerce. Some of the best and most beautiful essential oils available are distilled by women. Women generally have a better sense of smell than men and are better equipped to be creative in the interface of rational and intuitive conclusions for those in need of healing.

These developments find powerful expressions. I observed a most inspiring and uplifting example at the last World Congress of Medicinal and Aromatic Plants for Human Welfare. As the congress drew to a close and became ready to draw up its final recommendations for furthering and protecting the benefits humans can draw from medicinal plants, women professors from Brazil left indelible impressions on me. While conducting some of the most interesting research at their home universities on antineoplastic effects of sesquiterpenes and many other topics of sesquiterpene pharmacology, they also acted with great compassion to extend the meaning of human welfare from drug-manufacturers and their customers to *all* humans. Staunchly and calmly they did not relent until appropriate language was adopted calling for the protection of the rights of indigenous people—who share their knowledge about plants and usually have their intellectual property ripped off with no compensation—and the adoption of the necessary environmental measures. These women gave the much needed example that scientific research, when performed by women, can maintain a human face, can embody and include respect and protection for the earth and indigenous people, and can do this while concentrating on essential oils and their incredible healing powers.

Small is beautiful

Aromatherapy is still small and beautiful, both in the size of its shops and its overall sales. The human element, with all its beauty and imperfection, is very much intact in aromatherapy. As enterprises grow bigger the economic interest takes on a life of its own and the original product or service matters less and less. These ideas have been outlined in Schumacher's *Small is Beautiful,* a book I highly recommend to anyone interested in aromatherapy.

Aromatherapy does not have corporate superstructures, and owner-operated aromatherapy businesses do not need to create profit for shareholders. So even if some of the entrepreneurs in aromatherapy were less than perfect, they would still offer more healing for the buck. The difference lies in the joy of aromatherapy itself, not just financial rewards.

The true rewards of aromatherapy are found in a gradual change of lifestyle in which health can be maintained without drugs. Whenever essential oils are used, a large number of simultaneous processes create a powerful synergy. Wafting aromas stir our consciousness into initiating a reconnection with nature as well as lost archaic pieces of ourselves. Pieces of our identity and being that were lost as two hundred years of modern scientific conditioning separated our way of life from nature can be regained. Physical and emotional survival, on a sustainable basis, is only possible by following the laws of nature. The seeming contradictions to this—patients existing on chemotherapy, dialysis, and a regimen of thirty pills daily—can more aptly be viewed a sublethal existence that expresses the resilience of life in the face of overwhelming disease. To maintain this process of renewal, it is helpful to understand the ways in which essential oils and plants interact with human consciousness.

Essential oils and consciousness

In 1988 Daniel Pénoël presented his concept of the aromatic triptych. In this design he explained the action of essential oils in terms of the universe's basic components: matter, energy, and information. The "information age" has become a household term. The concept of information is the basis of the biggest global economic sector, and its nature an increasingly relevant topic in contemporary physics and cosmology. Scientists arrived at the conclusion that the ultimate source, origin, or substrate of everything has to be abstract. Matter and energy cannot exist without information. While information can be technical, it also guides our sensory perceptions, transmission of feelings, and intuitive recognition.[6]

The spectrum of information that interacts with and/or forms human consciousness is quite broad. Essential oils (in the context of aromatherapy) influence human consciousness in all layers of this very broad spectrum of relations and differences. A hierarchical system of the layers of consciousness that structure this spectrum of information has been developed. It is a key to this study and serves well to structure the qualitative diversity of benefits that constitute aromatherapy.

The material plane

The material plane comprises all manifestations of matter and the world that can be perceived with the senses. In the world of essential oils this includes molecular makeup, chemical qualities, and the way oils can be analyzed. Science has been very successful in elucidating the relations in the material world and describes them with, for instance, the laws of physics. Conventional pharmacology manifests itself in the material plane. When a drug manufactured in the lab according to the laws of physics and chemistry is given to a patient, a material change such as a drop in blood pressure, a rise in trace minerals, or a change in hormone levels can be measured. Scientific studies demonstrate the effectiveness of essential oils in the material plane.

The vital plane

The vital plane is comprised of manifestations of life such as language, behavior, instincts, reflexes, and emotions. Much of this biological programming is contained in our genetic code and in the older parts of the brain. With essential oils the vital plane is represented in our relation to odor, its influences on emotions, and how these factors contribute to a biological identity. Aromatherapy allows an expression of many of these vital instincts and reflexes, such as maternal instinct. Mothers who turn to aromatherapy as a health care modality for their families are not operating in the material plane but through natural instinct—the vital plane. This plane of consciousness, the expression of everything vital, has been correlated fittingly with male and female characteristics in Greek mythology through Asklepios, the god of medicine, and his daughter Hygieia, the goddess of healing.

The mental plane

On the mental plane we interact by making concepts, such as trying to understand or relate to one another. The mental plane is the first one that allows a choice between natural and synthetic, environmentally friendly or destructive, pill or oil. From the mental plane it is possible to connect to the biological and material, exercising influence on processes in these areas and understanding them. This plane is represented, for example, by a mental activity to optimize distillation processes, make choices about oil quality, understand pharmacology, or create an oil system that relates to yin and yang. Phenomena of thought and recognition are not identical with biological processes in the brain, which belong in the areas of matter and biology.

With these three "levels of consciousness" established, the influences that an oil can exert on the whole being can be more precisely described. When an oil interacts with a human being, the thalamus separates the event into three different impulses: one that reaches the motoric physical center (corresponding to the material plane of consciousness), one to the cortex (mental plane), and one to the hypothalamus (vital plane), which gives every event an emotional tint.[7] Instinct, biological programs, physical body, thought, and memory are all involved. The interaction on these three planes are qualitatively different from each other and are strictly hierarchical. The higher plane determines what goes on in the lower plane. For instance, while oil molecules have distinct properties, it is the vital aspects of the plant that determines what happens with oil, whether it is produced at all in the plant, stored in a plant oil

Table 9.1

Planes of reality	Planes of consciousness	Essential oil
God or corresponding concepts	Spiritual, traditional ritual and religious use corresponds to the interaction of myrrh compounds with receptor sites in the brain.	Myrrh
Soul	Psychosocial	St. Johnswort heals depression. Essential oils in general improve ego strength and reduce emotional lability.
Law, mathematics	Mental, reason, intellect	Basil stimulates mental activity.
Instinct, language	Vital	Bay laurel supports vital functions, such as the lymphatic system.
Molecules, planets	Material	Everlast, pronounced physical effects.

container, or released into the air for plant or insect communication or self-defense. These processes are not determined by matter itself but by the higher biological/vital plane. "Holistic" means that not just a symptom or a disease should be recognized but the whole person (what may work for one individual can be inappropriate for another and vice versa). Humans are not simply a physical body with parts and functions; interaction with the higher biological and mental expressions of our being is important. Pharmacology—medicine as a science—by its own admission operates exclusively on the material plane (science tries to eliminate any vital parameters, as they are too hard to control). What distinguishes aromatherapy the most from conventional medicine is the vertical flow of information from plants to humans through all planes of consciousness, not just the material.

The psychosocial plane

The relationship of humans with each other as well as to nature has been marginalized in the technological age. The corresponding fourth plane of consciousness (the psychosocial plane) was fully neglected by the materialistic worldview—with dire consequences for the well-being of the soul. On this plane of consciousness human needs are fulfilled that cannot be satisfied by the three lower planes, such as the desire to be kind, to have friends, and to live in a morally and ethically satisfying environment. There is still evidence in small, noncorporate aroma businesses for acceptance of the psychosocial plane. Respect for other humans and nature is still inherent in the field. Of course, material gain and the desire for power are also present. But in aromatherapy, economics and ethics do not necessarily compete but are still connected to some degree, strikingly different from the world of big medicine. Doing business while maintaining respect for nature is an expression of the psychosocial plane and makes aromatherapy a forerunner of the economic trend of the future. And what may be viewed as most amazing is that controlled, double-blind psychological tests were performed in the seventies that clearly demonstrate the effectiveness and interaction of essential oils and their components with the phenomena of the soul. Four weeks of therapy brought significant improvements in such areas as restlessness, unexplainable nervousness, hot flashes, and headaches. These are all symptoms typical of autonomic nervous system imbalances. But more fascinating is the fact that patients also experienced highly significant improvements in such conditions of the soul as ego strength, irritability, and emotional stability. The relevance of plant healing for the fourth plane of consciousness—the psychosocial plane—is harder to discover. It begins with the responsibility for health outside of oneself: one's family and friends.

The spiritual plane

Well-being of the soul does not result from the self realization of the lower planes but from the subordination to the higher ones. This leads directly to the highest plane of consciousness, the spiritual plane. Humans need spirituality in their lives. And while science may deem it superstition, Leandis believes that "only the spirit is real, more than anything you ever encounter in this life."[8]

Pharmaceutical medicine feeds only one plane of human consciousness. In contrast, essential oils give us glimpses of the higher planes via their specific interaction with the vital fields of odor, emotion, and identity. Essential oils remind us of the wonders of creation. Plant medicine drinks from a fountain that has a missing ingredient:

Inakelinya, a spiritual elder of the Kuna Indians in Panama, says as much: "In the bath with the plants, there is contact with more than just the wisdom of the plants, there is contact with the spirits. They don't touch you, but they talk to you. You can hear them talking to you. When you get one of these baths your mind opens and the power of the plants comes through you."[9]

We can use our mental powers to contemplate all aspects of our interaction with plants, from evolutionary development of their essential-oil molecules to the ritualistic and divinatory use of fragrances in other cultures. Essential oils form the basis for a healing modality that fully transcends the old scientific-materialistic paradigm but is still easily accessible to Western industrialized societies. Essential oils offer healing, maintain well-being, stimulate spiritual exploration, and are morally desirable—their production is sustainable rather than exploitative, and they tend not to be cruelly tested on animals as most conventional medicines are.

Conclusions based on the belief that all aspects of human life can be explained through the understanding of the mental plane lead invariably to what in contemporary computer lingo is called a system error. Such a mistake would occur if one tried to analyze the cultural and historical meaning of frankincense in Christianity with the laws of molecular biology. Errors like this are common.

Chronic fatigue, probably a problem of the mental plane, is nonetheless exclusively approached by the old paradigm with the means and tools of the material plane. Psychology attempts to explain the problems of the soul—the fourth or psychological plane—with science, or, in other words, with the tools of the lower three levels of consciousness. Not surprisingly, psychology has been made a substitute religion by somehow adjusting the hierarchy of consciousness to the needs of psychology.

Guidance in the search for the realities of the spirit is found in the knowledge of North American Indians for whom the connection of plants to the power of spirit is entirely clear. One such Native, Leandis, writes, "You've got to reconnect with your soul. If you don't it will kill you. Your problem is not physical, could become, it's your soul. Your soul can effect the physical." Telisforo, an Indian elder from the Talamanca Mountains in Panama, writes, "Nobody has worked medicine without God. It is a lie if someone tells you it works without God." Hermengildo and Tomas Aguilar—Cabecar Indians of Panama—believe that plants possess spirituality:

> When we gather the herbs, we talk to them as we pull them up from the land. We take them into our hands, and we know inside the herb is a good spirit. The plants have a spirit, a good spirit, and we talk to them. We know the good spirit will help us with our family and with the people we are going to cure. The good spirits will take out the illnesses that people have inside their bodies. We know there are many people who have lost their way. They don't understand spiritual things. We know that evil spirits are inside the person who is sick. The herb will help them. So many look at the plants and see only grass and weeds. They are blind. They have made themselves blind and closed themselves off from their connection with God.[10]

The medicine of aromatherapy and essential oils is part of the original creation (synthetic drugs are the manifestation of the material/scientific plane). Plants connect to the spirit. For everyone caught in the realization of the lower three levels and wanting to escape, plants have the power to provide the missing element for healing the soul.

Similar conclusions are reached by E. F. Schumacher:

> I have tried to show what these ideas are likely to be today: a total denial of meaning and purpose of human existence on earth, leading to the total despair of anyone who really believes in them. Fortunately, as I said, the heart is often more intelligent than the mind and refuses to accept these ideas in their full weight. So the man is saved from despair, but landed in confusion. His fundamental convictions are confused; hence his actions, too, are confused and uncertain. If he would only allow the light of consciousness to fall on the centre and face the question of his fundamental convictions, he could create order where there is disorder. That would "educate" him, in the sense of leading him out of the darkness of his metaphysical confusion. I do not think, however, that this can be successfully done unless he quite consciously accepts—even only provisionally—a number of metaphysical ideas which are almost directly opposite to the ideas (stemming from the nineteenth century) that have lodged in his mind. I shall mention three examples. While the nineteenth century ideas deny or obliterate the hierarchy of levels in the universe, the notion of an hierarchical order is an indispensable instrument of understanding. Without the recognition of "levels of being" or "grades of significance" we cannot make the world intelligible to ourselves nor have we the slightest possibility to define our own position, the position of man, in the scheme of the universe. It is only when we can see the world as a ladder, and when we can see man's position on the ladder, that we can recognize a meaningful task for man's life on earth. Maybe it is man's task—or simply, if you like, man's happiness—to attain a higher degree of realization of his potentialities, a higher level of being or "grade of significance" than that which comes to him "naturally": We cannot even study this possibility except by recognizing the existence of a hierarchical structure. To the extent that we interpret the world through the great, vital ideas of the nineteenth century, we are blind to these differences of level, because we have been blinded.[11]

As soon, however, as we accept the existence of "levels of being," we can readily understand, for instance, why the methods of physical science cannot explain the benefits of plants or why the findings of physics—as Einstein recognized—have no philosophical implications.

"Do you think you can take over the universe and improve it? I do not believe it can be done."
—Tao Te Ching

TEN

Essential Oils

According to the International Organization for Standardization, an essential oil is a "product obtained from natural raw material, either by distillation with water and steam, or from the epicarp of citrus fruits by mechanical processing, or by dry distillation. The essential oil is subsequently separated from the aqueous phase by physical means."[1] From a technical standpoint, that is a very useful definition of essential oils. Additionally, there is a great deal of literature available describing how essential oils are made and what the intricacies of the harvesting process are.[2] For example, proceedings of the annual International Symposium on Essential Oils published between 1976 and 1985 present the relevant research regarding the plants' essential oils occurrence, physiology, and composition of essential oils.

For the scope of therapeutic aromatherapy, it should be added that essential oils must be truly natural, because only genuine oils convey a whole and complex set of signs and the complete information from the plant.

The distillation of essential oils and fragrant waters from plants is one of the oldest skills of humanity. The famous Mohenjo Daro distillation apparatus from Afghanistan dates back to the year 3000 B.C. and is presumed to be the oldest.[3] Arab science was brought to Europe between the eleventh and thirteenth centuries, mainly through the intellectual centers of the time founded at Toledo, Spain, and the School of Salerno, one of the principle ports of call during the Crusades. From there, techniques such as distillation became known in the south of France, particularly in the region of Montpelier. Until the Middle Ages, distillation was performed for the preparation of aromatic waters; the oily liquids floating on top of the distillates were often discarded as undesirable by-products! The first description of the distillation of a true essential oil was given by a Catalonian physician, Arnold de Villanova (1235–1311), whose essences were included in the pharmacopoeias of the time. Paracelsus, a doctor from the fifteenth century, called essential oils the "quinta essenzia" of the plant (roughly translated as "creating the essence to the fifth degree"), and in 1500 and 1507, Brunschwig, a physician from Strasbourg, France, published his two famous volumes on distillation entitled *"Liber de Arte Destillandi."*[4]

Steam distillation

The process of steam distillation of essential oils is relatively simple when described in terms of the evaporation and subsequent condensation of two immiscible liquids. Upon heating, when the vapor pressures of the two phases of water and oil accumulate, their sum equals atmospheric pressure, the heterogeneous mixture of water and oil begins to boil. This view has been challenged by E. F. K. Denny, longtime director of The Bridestowe Estate and Lavender Plantation in Tasmania. He suggests that the heat of condensation of droplets of steam condensing on a leaf or plant material is the relevant parameter that determines the evaporation and distillation of an essential oil.

The origin of essential oils from the plant metabolism, and their production by the steam distillation process in its many variations, has been described in detail in the literature. Comprehensive accounts are found in *Essential Oils*, by Gildemeister and Hoffmann, and *Essential Oils* by Guenther. While these encyclopedic texts view essential oils mainly as raw materials for industrial use (fragrance and flavor), the 1956 edition of the Gildemeister and Hoffman also contains an extensive and highly informative section on essential-oil pharmacology.

Quality and purity

A comprehensive enumeration of quality considerations for essential oils intended for therapeutic use was introduced in a much overlooked *Huiles Essentielles - Hydrolates - Distillation, Qualité, Contrôle de la Pureté, Indications Majeures,* by Henri Viaud, in 1983. Viaud's criteria for the quality requirements of essential oils for therapeutic use mark the first time where the wholeness and the unaltered natural composition of an essential oil was given absolute priority over more technical considerations such as active ingredients or potential variation in composition. Natural variation is seen as a valid expression of nature, not an impediment to manufacturing and commerce.

Contemporary thinking is often influenced by the current competitive way of doing business, in which quality, price, and origin are considered. But for applications of personal healing it is wiser to stick with a supplier of essential oils that are known to work. Purchasing an oil from another supplier who buys from different sources seems less recommendable in light of the many variables that will be different and may influence the healing power of the oil. It helps to think of genuine and authentic essential oils the same way we think of fine wines. A Mouton Rothschild cabernet of a given vintage has a distinct identity and cannot be substituted with a cabernet from another part of the world. This identity is best reflected with another vintage of Mouton. This is also true for essential oils—their healing characteristics are more predictable when the oils are chosen from the same geographical location, and, better still, the same producer.

Over the years, the quality criteria outlined by Viaud have virtually become the standard in all areas of holistic and therapeutic

Table 10.1: Average annual production of essential oils and related fragrance materials listed by oil, extraction type, and metric tons produced annually

Low volume (high price)			**Medium volume (medium price)**			**High volume (low price)**		
Ambrette Sd	B,E	0.5	Bergamot	E	115	Cedarwood (USA)	E	1640
Black currant	C	0.9	Clary sage	E	45	Cedarwood (China)	E	450
Cistus	E	2	Geranium	E	130	Citronella	E	2300
Chamo., Ger.	E	8	Guaiac wood	E	60	Clove bud	E	2000
Galbanum	E,R	12	Lavender	E,C	200	Corn mint	E	2100
Jasmine	C	11	Oakmoss	C	50	Eucalyptus (cineole)	E	1400
Myrrh	E,R	4	Patchouli	E	500	Eucalyptus (citronellal)	E	1700
Narcissus	C	1	Sandal-wood	E	70	Lavandin	C,E	900
Neroli	E	1	Tree moss	C,R	110	Peppermint	E	2200
Olibanum	E,R	4	Vetiver	E	260	Spearmint	E	1400
Opoponax	E,R	3	Ylang ylang	E	87			
Orange flwr	C	1.5						
Orris	B,R	3.5						
Rose	C,E	15						
Tuberose	C	0.6						
Violet leaf	C	0.2						

Abbreviations: C=concrete; **R**=resinold; **E**=essential oil; **B**=butter
Source: *Perfumes: Art, Science & Technology,* PM Müller and D. Lamparsky, Elsevier Applied Science, New York, 1991.

aromatherapy. Because essential oils are altered not only by the addition of foreign matter but also with materials of natural origin (such as other essential oils), certain terminology was adopted to exclude the latter "soft" manipulations. Following are Viaud's requirements for essential oils to be considered genuine and authentic.

During all stages of producing a genuine and authentic oil the final goal should be to produce the best possible essential oil. The distillation of these oils is carried out as slowly and carefully as possible. Distilling genuine and authentic oils from wild plants additionally requires that the workers harvesting the plants be knowledgeable and honest in gathering only plants from the one species to be distilled.

Genuine and authentic oils should be distilled slowly and, if necessary, at reduced pressure and temperature. A lower distillation temperature protects the essences from being oxidized, and fragile molecules from being destroyed by excessive temperature. Yet distillation at low pressure and temperature inevitably takes longer.

"Genuine" means absolutely unaltered. This means the addition of even natural substances is not permitted. Genuine essential oils should be:

- *100% natural:* This means no synthetic esters, emulsifying agents, petrol-based diluents such as mineral oil, dipropyleneglycol, phtalates, or any other synthetic additive.
- *100% pure:* No similar essential oils may be added. For example, lavender is often extended with hybrid species called lavandins to create the oil.
- *100% complete:* Oils shall not be decolorized, recolored, or deterpenated. In the perfume and food industries, the use of deterpenated essences is very common (for example, citrus-juice concentrates). However, deterpenating essences for aromatherapy results in lower bioactivity and may even make them more toxic.

"Authentic" means that the oil should reflect the composition of the plant specified on the label, not a mix of plants that go by the same name or that may grow alongside the actual plant being harvested. Essential oils must be distilled from plants or their parts that belong only to one clearly identified species. Two essences with different compositions have different effects, and their potential healing qualities are likely to be different. It is, therefore, necessary to characterize essential oils precisely.

Analysis shows that the chemical composition of an essential oil is generally quite constant within a botanical species. Conditions of climate or harvest effect nuances of its composition, but usually not to such an extent that it becomes an entirely different oil.

Chemotypes

Sometimes the designation of a so-called chemotype is necessary, such as when plants of one botanical species produce essential oils of distinctly different chemical compositions. Important examples of this phenomenon are the essential oils of rosemary and thyme. For example, three chemotypes of rosemary *(Rosmarinus officinalis)* are commonly distinguished as follows:

1. *Rosmarinus officinalis,* camphor-borneol type (Spain, Croatia)
2. *Rosmarinus officinalis,* 1,8-cineole type (Tunisia, Morocco)
3. *Rosmarinus officinalis,* verbenone type (Corsica)

Due to their different compositions, these oils can be applied for various purposes.

Up to six or seven chemotypes of thyme *(Thymus vulgaris)* are commonly distinguished. Among them:

1. *Thymus vulgaris,* linalool type
2. *Thymus vulgaris,* geraniol type
3. *Thymus vulgaris,* thujanol-4 type
4. *Thymus vulgaris,* thymol type
5. *Thymus vulgaris,* carvacrol type

Methods used to analyze essential oils

Essential oils are commonly analyzed by either gas chromatography (GC) or a combination of gas chromatography and mass spectroscopy (GC-MS). GC and GC-MS are powerful methods for routine analysis, quality control, and research. Because of varying parameters such as different machines, columns, flow rates, temperature programs, and so on, chromatograms can usually only be compared within one experimental setting. Usefulness of the chromatogram is, therefore, limited to those performing the analysis. It appears that analysis of essential oils by gas chromatography (and GC-MS) will remain largely irrelevant to the end-consumer and to the retailer, which means the end-user must simply trust in the truthfulness of a certificate of purity issued by an independent laboratory. Such a certificate does not necessarily mean that the essential oils are pure as claimed. The odds are there is as much fluff involved in certificates of purity as in the sales talk of an essential-oil distributor. The recent increased emphasis on chromatograms mostly reflects clever playing by a vendor, who knows that the public is more likely to believe something once a machine is involved.

Why would anyone advertise essential oils as being of mediocre quality or less than the very best? Quite naturally, vendors offer "only the best" and, as a result, such claims have become utterly meaningless.

For someone seriously involved in aromatherapy, it is almost imperative to understand the possibilities of modern analytical techniques that are routinely utilized to analyze essential oils. As commonly understood, temperature-programmed gas chromatography is a method well-suited for a quick assessment of the quality of essential oils.

> Characterization of the quality of an essential oil by determining the concentration of main constituent (for example, eucalyptole, 1,8-cineole in eucalyptus oil) is absolutely insufficient to properly assess the quality or the origin of an essential oil. This may be obvious, but must be pointed out since many of the requirements set forth by the

> pharmacopoeias of different countries are based on that type of assessment. As far as the pharmacopoeia is concerned, a synthetic substitute fulfills the quality requirement for an essential oil as well as the natural original. Kubeczka continues, "Quality assessment must not be the determination of one main component, but has to take into account the secondary and trace constituents. This obviously leads to many different and very specialized examinations."[5]

To establish identity and origin of an essential oil it is necessary to employ a method that allows for the identification and quantification of all constituents of an essential oil with sufficient selectivity, exactness, and reproducibility. For basic quality control of essential oils, gas chromatography can satisfy many of these demands.

A chromatographic method separates the different components in an essential oil. The resulting printout, in which substances are recorded as peaks, is called a "chromatogram." The gas chromatography's usefulness is dependent on the availability of other chromatograms for comparison and reference. Gas chromatography itself does not identify the substance that causes a given peak—identifications are made by comparing with a standard. If the known test substance (standard) appears at the same spot as the peak in a chromatogram, identity is assumed.

Given the complexity of essential-oil compositions, such identifications are often ambiguous and spectroscopic methods must be used to identify a component with precision. This has become easier with the advent of machines that perform a "mass-spectrum" of the isolated substances immediately after they leave the GC. They perform a dual operation in one box: First the essential oil is separated by gas chromatography. Then the isolated components are, one by one, identified via separate (mass) spectra. There is one spectrum for every compound. Interpretation of mass-spectra, however, is not trivial and is mainly done by computerized reference libraries. Interpretation is, therefore, a question of the quality of the available libraries. In real life, this means that big research entities that specialize in fragrance research own very impressive libraries of the mass-spectra of fragrance materials. Such libraries represent great value, and such data tends to be proprietary. This also means that the computerized evaluation of a GC-MS from a lab that has not previously specialized in this type of analysis will probably not yield very satisfying results.

In principle, this is also true for gas chromatography alone. A lab that specializes in essential-oil GC will have the reference materials to produce useful analyses of essential oils. Experts familiar with essential oils chromatograms will spot unusual components or gross adulterants immediately.

Gas chromatography has its greatest value for the producer who can use it to determine if the oil of this year's crop has the same or similar composition as last year's harvest. Isolated gas chromatograms attached to one essential oil—mostly produced by the original producer in France—have only limited significance because it is practically impossible for the layperson to verify the interpretation of the chromatogram. These chromatograms represent no practical value to someone not involved in interpreting them.[5]

As a result, we can say that gas chromatography is useful but by itself has only limited value to prove essential oil purity because conclusions can only be made through comparison with corresponding reference materials. Conversely, if a standard way of referencing results of GC is desired, the report should clearly state *who* performed the analysis (an independent lab or the manufacturer) and *who* interpreted the chromatogram (a qualified expert or the lab technician of the manufacturer). The involvement of isolated chromatograms to support purity of an essential-oil product without any other specification is misleading. Furthermore, the requirements of correct sampling must be considered; it is one thing to present a chromatogram and another to be reasonably sure that the analyzed sample is representative of a given product.

Chromatography

Chromatographic methods are employed to separate mixtures of chemical compounds into isolated substances. They are used analytically, such as in gas chromatography, to obtain information about the characteristics of a composition. They are also used to purify or isolate a desired material from unwanted substances that may be mixed with it. In a chemical synthesis, the desired substance is almost always mixed with undesired by-products; preparative chromatography can be used to separate the desired material from the undesired by-products and residues. Most commonly used are:

- *Gas chromatography (GC).* Gas chromatography is commonly employed for routine quality checks on essential oils. Mixtures are separated while they are carried through capillary columns by a carrier gas.
- *High performance liquid chromatography (HPLC).* This very powerful method is used to separate hard-to-separate mixtures and is very useful for essential-oil analysis. HPLC utilizes liquids under pressure as opposed to a gas-flowing phase.
- *Gel liquid chromatography (GLC).* In gel liquid chromatography, substances are separated while flowing through a column packed with porous gel. This method is slow and the results are variable. It is not normally used for essential-oil analysis.
- *Thin layer chromatography (TLC).* This method has very good separation power. Here the mixtures become separated by rising up along a thin layer of silica. In practical use this method is mainly for the analysis of tinctures and extracts and only to a limited degree for essential-oil analysis.

Spectroscopy

The aim of spectroscopic methods is to observe certain physical properties of a given substance in order to gather clues about its chemical structure. In specific cases, these methods can also be employed to detect impurities when it is possible to observe a physical property that is unique to an adulterant.

- *Infrared spectroscopy (IR).* A single compound (or a mixture) is subjected to a spectrum of infrared light (light with wavelengths ranging between two and fifteen microns). Certain structural features of a molecule (such as a ketone group) will cause absorption of infrared light of a specific wavelength. The resulting readout is called an IR Spectrum. Absorption of light with wavelengths around six microns is associated with ketone groups. The spectrum will very clearly reflect the ketone group. It is, however, more involved and often impossible to determine the complete structure of a molecule by IR alone.
- *Ultraviolet spectroscopy (UV).* Ultraviolet spectroscopy works along the same principles as IR spectroscopy. However, the absorption of wavelengths in the ultraviolet range (200–350 nanometers) is measured. This technique is of limited importance for essential-oil analysis in general.
- *Nuclear magnetic resonance (NMR) 1H-NMR and 13C-NMR.* These are spectroscopic methods that measure magnetic parameters of the indicated nuclei (either 1H or 13C). An extremely powerful tool for structure elucidation in a research situation is 13C-NMR. These methods are too involved for use as a tool for the quality control of essential oils.
- *Mass spectrometry (MS).* Molecules are subjected to high-energy electrons and burst into pieces. Mass spectrometry records the masses of all the different fragments into which the molecule bursts. The exact path of fragmentation (the sequence of decreasing masses into which the molecule decays) is for all practical purposes unique for every molecule. Mass spectrometry allows almost unambiguous identification of chemical structures. Consequently, competent interpretation of unknown mass spectra is highly involved and time-consuming. In combination with GC (GC-MS) it is a very powerful, complex, and expensive tool for essential-oil research. This method is mainly used by universities and for corporate research.
- *Enantio-selective gas chromatography (ESGC) and isotope ratio*

mass-spectrometry (IRMS). These two analytical methods allow for some of the best assessment of authenticity of essential oils. Many of the most common molecules occurring in essential oils are "chiral," meaning they exist in two enantiomeric forms. Natural essential oils are characterized by distinctive patterns; for instance, in monoterpene hydrocarbons this is seen in the distribution of their plus or minus enantiomeric forms. The enantiomeric ratio of constituents of essential oils of the same species but of different origins is similar but not identical. If the specific enantiomeric ratio for a plant essential oil is known, adulterations of essential oils with compounds emanating from the laboratory (racemic compounds) can be detected. IRMS utilizes another endogenous parameter of biosynthesis to ascertain authenticity of an oil or an oil component. When plants photosynthesize, they distinguish carbon dioxide from the common carbon isotope and carbon dioxide molecules with a heavier isotope. Organically bound carbon is deficient in heavier isotopes compared to the carbon dioxide in the air. This deficit is not identical for all plants but is dependent on its type of photosynthesis. The ratio of carbon isotopes in essential oils or their components is often specific for a given plant, and these different ratios can be utilized to distinguish between substances of synthetic and natural origin as well as between substances of different natural origins.

"Organic" French lavender

Analysis of lavender oils on the market is an interesting project. Every supplier would like to carry the best possible lavender, as it is a staple in aromatherapy. The characteristic of the desired French lavender is a high content of the ester, linalyl acetate. This requirement has led to many attempts to adjust the ester content upward, from spraying linalyl acetate onto the plants right before harvest to the simple elongation of lavender oil with synthetic or semisynthetic linalool and linalyl acetate.

In a gas chromatogram, synthetic linalool and linalyl acetate will appear at the same spot as their natural counterparts, making it virtually impossible for even the initiated wholesaler or layperson to recognize this kind of adulteration. Obviously, it is in the interest of the aromatherapist to receive true, unadulterated lavender oil, especially when it is billed as such! Following is an outline of how the addition of synthetic linalool and linalyl acetate can be identified via GC-MS.

According to the literature, the combined contents of linalool and linalyl acetate in true lavender oil should reach an upper limit of 70 percent. Consequently, oils with combined linalool/linalyl acetate contents of up to 80 percent are quite suspect.

Synthetic linalool and linalyl acetate are contaminated with small amounts of by-products from their synthesis, among them is dihydro linalool and dihydro linalyl acetate. In a gas chromatogram, these target compounds may show up either as minute peaks, making up a tiny fraction of the whole oil, or they may be hidden underneath much larger peaks of other components and thus remain virtually undetected. Target compounds can be detected with gas chromatography coupled with mass spectrometry and selective ion mass spectrometry (SIMS). Since the target compounds form ions with masses that are known to differ from the natural compounds by two units, one can selectively search for ions with these masses and, by identifying these contamination products, prove the addition of synthetic linalool and/or linalyl acetate.

The commercial reality

"For every activity there is a certain appropriate scale, and the more active and intimate the activity, the smaller the number of people that can take part... What scale is appropriate? It depends on what we are trying to do. The question of scale is extremely crucial today, in political, social and economic affairs just as in almost everything else... The really serious matters of life cannot be calculated. We cannot directly calculate what is right , but we jolly well know what is wrong." —E. F. Schumacher.

These considerations bring up questions relating to the nature and size of essential-oil production when the purpose of the oils is healing. Two main approaches can be identified: the eclectic, self-medicating or practicing professional who will only work with genuine oils and accepts lapses in supply (and who accepts realistic prices that allow the producer to survive), and the aromatherapy entrepreneur who dreams of skyrocketing sales.

If essential oils are intended for healing, they must relate to the framework in which healing can happen, and healing cannot be scaled-up much. True healing may not even be scaled-up past a one-on-one interaction.

An evaluation of the current essential-oil supply reveals that those oils that really contain the magic and are unaltered without exception are supplied by small companies who themselves buy from small or mid-sized producers. When companies grow big, the requirements of continued supply, smooth distribution, cash flow, and so on take on a life of their own. If a company is honest, the original goal to heal gives way to the simpler desire to provide trendy and gifty bath products.

If the demand for oils increases, it may exceed the volume that established sources can supply. Keeping up a supply of genuine and authentic oils is difficult when demand skyrockets. This is not to say that there are not enough of these oils available around the globe, quite the opposite is true. The recent past has seen many entrances into the market of essential oils intended for aromatherapy. Nonetheless, to maintain integrity an importer would have to remain in contact with many small enterprises and be willing to deal with the administrative hurdles involved in importing from developing nations (customs clearance, freight rates, delays in communication, difficulties in financial transfers, and so on).

As a result, the original drive of an operator—to search out the best oils and maintain passion for travel and research—gives way to more streamlined principles of organizing. In the interest of an uninterrupted supply of the goods to be sold, one turns in all likelihood to the big import houses that provide essential oils for industrial usage. But the import houses make their money by processing the oil. The sad consequence is that too many oils today come from the processing plant. These are typically not synthetics, but are factory-mixed natural components (isolated from the oils of other plants), semisynthetics (a natural substance altered by a chemical reaction), and fragrance. Such oils are raw materials for fragrance products intended for the mass-market. For healing based on the interaction of plant substance with humans they are next to useless, because diversity and complexity of the plant has been substituted with cost-effective industrial surrogates.

Processed oils are often self-evident by their unrealistically low price, achieved by clever manipulations much like the fast-food burger for ninety-nine cents. Large brokerage firms typically offer essential oils at prices below the original production cost—for example, one pound of rosemary essential oil for just under eight dollars. This is a clear indication of industrial meddling. In light of this reality, the fretting about oil quality that occurs among competing suppliers in the aromatherapy industry has degenerated into a boring exchange of marketing hype. Naturally every supplier sells "only the best" quality oils, even if they do originate in big processing warehouses in New York.

Orange oil

The implications of size play themselves out with almost shocking clarity with the case of orange oil. Commercial orange oil from large-scale citrus plantations is almost invariably tainted with intolerably high concentrations of known and unknown pesticides. This is a direct result of the lack of biological diversity in huge citrus monocultures, which become extremely susceptible to infestation and virtually could not exist without heavy doses of pesticides. A new situation has arisen for the supply of orange oil in Israel. Chlorinated polycyclic pesticides have been outlawed in that country and citrus-peel oils originating from there are, therefore, free of those pesticides. Outlawing DDT and Lindan, however, does not mean that *all* pesticides have been outlawed, nor does it mean that the citrus is organically grown. As you might expect, there are suppliers who confuse (semi) pesticide-free with "organic."

True, organic orange oil of exquisite fullness is produced, according to biodynamic agriculture, by Demeter-certified farms in southern Europe. For aromatherapy, they represent a much higher value than the previously described ones. These orange oils are useless for any large-scale business, but they are quite useful to small-scale aromatherapy companies that have healing as their focus.

Standards

The creation of quality standards for essential oils used for aromatherapy has been perceived by many to be a solution to the aforementioned problems. The odds are, it is not. Essential oils may be impossible to standardize because they reflect the intrinsic variability of nature. Standards existing in the past were interpreted by processors as license to adjust the oil to fit the standard. This has been useful for the manufacture of products with exactly reproducible quality for the mass-market. But holistic healing requires unprocessed oils.

For this very reason, attempts to standardize essential oils to fit a certain set of ingredients seem counterproductive. Essential oils should be as rich and complex as they are when they come out of the still. Seasonal or yearly variations (or variations originating from different distillation processes) should be permitted because they are the legitimate expression of the regional geographic and climatic influences as well as the interaction of the grower with nature in crafting the oil. The human way of making an oil (as opposed to that of gigantic agribusiness), corresponds with the scope of healing—a human activity that cannot be scaled-up at will. Variable and complex essential oils present drawbacks for smooth exploitation by large businesses but are less problematic for aromatherapy.

Oils produced for holistic aromatherapy are not starting materials. They are end-products made by real people by way of agriculture rather than chemical processes. Consequently, such oils are more expensive than their mass-produced cousins. Despite the higher prices for genuine oils, holistic aromatherapy is still economically competitive because very little goes a long way.

While many businesses continue to prosper by securing success in the mass-market, this strategy brings endless compromise and insures mediocrity. In the long run, success is not defined by this type of marketing but by the excellence of a product and a living craft. McDonald's is certainly "successful" as a food-processing business, but so is the excellent restaurant in a small town that only locals know about. To extend the analogy, processed oils, in feel and effect, are much like processed foods. At a certain point, processed foods only marginally resemble the flavors, aromas, and textures of the real thing. The local restaurant, however, strives to put food on the plate that represents and maybe even heightens the original textures, flavors, and aromas. That restaurant excels by producing quality, not maximizing output.

The fine-wine industry, which also deals in expensive liquids of varying natural origin, shows how a reliable standard of authenticity can be created and how it can be challenged by the demands of industrialization. There are vintners who make their wine with as little wine-*making* as possible—letting the wine reflect the earth on which it grows and the sunlight that ripens the fruit. Then there are big industrial reserve cabernets that are deliberately constructed to please the masses.

An analysis of wine is generally not performed to ascertain authenticity. A consumer purchasing a Robert Mondavi cabernet would never think of subjecting the bottle to a GC analysis to determine if it does or does not contain the juice of a cabernet grape. The consumer has good reason to trust that the name Mondavi guarantees the authenticity of the product in the bottle. The point to be made is that while analysis is absolutely critical in the field of holistic aromatherapy, the right approach is to not rely exclusively on technology and science but to integrate the human element.

This means creating an appreciation and awareness of the people who provide pure essential oils: the growers and distillers who raise a crop, produce an essential oil, and bring it to the market.

As the past vividly illustrates, keeping sources secret and hiding behind standards, analysis, pharmacopoeia, and national formularies have done nothing for the consumer. In the end, standards only benefit clever suppliers who use them to betray the consumer's trust. As a result of the progress in analytical technology, clever methods of reconstituting essential oils were developed. This is done by adjusting essential oils to the guidelines or standards set up in pharmacopoeia or formularies. This technique has developed to the point where essential oils are reconstituted as a whole. As a result, "natural" essential oils are mixed with reconstituted cousins made up of natural isolates that can be offered at a low price.

Competition from cheap, reconstituted oils causes growers and producers of *real* essential oils to be in a constant squeeze by primary purchasers not wanting to pay the prices that the growers and producers need to support their farms. Growers in France may find it expedient to discontinue growing lavender and turn their attention to more profitable cash crops such as cabbage. In essence, by pushing the price down on genuine oils (through reconstituted oils), we are putting a squeeze on the source of those materials that we are trying to acquire for aromatherapy. This does not make sense.

Procuring essential oils for healing purposes really is best done through companies that share the vision of a healing aromatherapy. The original intention of the enterprise effects the product. This means that parts of aromatherapy are capable of turning away from the seemingly irrepressible logic of modern-day economics—that more is better and that in order to grow, one must tolerate the accompanying inhumanity and environmental destruction. Genuine essential oils deliver what conventional medicine cannot: they manifest through intermediate technology and they spawn healing technologies similar to those of nature—noiseless, gentle, and effective.

"**No medicine cures what happiness cannot.**"
—Gabriel Garcia Marquez, *Of Love and Other Demons*

ELEVEN
Composition, Biosynthesis, and Safety of Essential Oils

From the first structure elucidation of terpenes by Otto Wallach, who deciphered the structural formula for pinene and camphene and similar terpenes, an enormous broadening of knowledge about the chemical composition of essential oils has occurred. In general, advances were slower in the beginning but have grown exponentially with the advent of instrumental analysis and its computerization. Consequently, the first chemical structures to become known were those that were present in essential oils in high percentages and/or were relevant to the fragrance industry.

At first, the analysis of terpenes progressed steadily and with many useful results. The determination of the chemical structure of the sesquiterpene compounds turned out to be much more cumbersome. One of the biggest obstacles was the separation of sesquiterpenes that were almost identical. Stereo chemical issues complicated the matter further. Today it is thought that approximately two hundred basic skeletal families of sesquiterpenes make up 99 percent of all sesquiterpenes found in essential oils. These basic structures are present in many variations. For example, in addition to caryophyllene, there exists isocaryophyllene, beta caryophyllene, caryophyllene epoxide, and caryophyllene oxide.

This is a general phenomenon; there are many different variations for every basic sesquiterpene structure. Because of the great similarity between many sesquiterpenes, even with today's sophisticated means of analysis and evaluation we are unable to simply put an essential oil into a GC-MS instrument and have the computer identify all of the different sesquiterpenes correctly. The high rate of inaccuracies in determining sesquiterpenes exactly through simple GC-MS analysis have been the object of scientific deliberations and warnings against trusting stand-alone GC-MS analysis.[1] Today approximately a thousand sesquiterpenes are known to occur in essential oils.

The biological origin of essential oils

The pharmacologically important plant constituents arise from the primary or secondary plant metabolism. The chemical reactions of the primary metabolism are, for the most part, identical for all plants. The end-products are nucleic acids, fats, proteins, carbohydrates, and so on. They are necessary for the plant as reserves and as sources of energy. These products are mainly used as base material, rarely as actual medicines. Exceptions are enzymes and castor oil.

The chemical reactions of the secondary metabolism are not necessarily vital for the plant. They can vary from species to species and are the expression of the chemical individuality of the plant organism. Some, such as essential oils, are stored in specifically equipped cells. These products have no significance as sources of energy and whether they have a physiological significance for the plant is often not entirely clear. However, some of those compounds are important for propagation and survival of the species. Most substances that are used as medicines are products of the secondary metabolism and are distinguished by very specific pharmacological properties.

Main components

Two basic biosynthetic pathways are responsible for almost 100 percent of all essential-oil constituents. Terpenes, sesquiterpenes, diterpenes, and triterpenes all are the products of the terpenoid or mevalogenic biosynthetic pathway. The other large group of components can be summarized as phenylpropanoids. They are by-products of the amino acid metabolism and share the amino acid phenyl alanine as the starting point of their synthesis.[2]

Table 11.1: Products of the mevalogenic biosynthetic pathway (terpenes and higher homologues)

Class of compounds	Number of isoprene units	Occurrence
Monoterpenes	2	Essential oil components, iridoids
Sesquiterpenes	3	Essential oil components
Diterpenes	4	Components of essential oils and resins, vitamin A, phytol, gibberellines
Triterpenes	6	Squalen, steroids, heart glycosides
Tetraterpenes	8	Carotenoids, xanthophylles
Polyterpenes	µ	caoutchouc, guttapercha

Compounds with ten carbon atoms (terpenes)

Geranyl-pyrophosphate is the biological precursor of the acyclic monoterpene alcohol, geraniol, from which acyclic terpenes such as citronellol, ocimene, or linalool are formed. Synthesis of terpene hydrocarbons primarily occurs in young plant material. The formation of oxygen-containing terpenes, secondary modifications, prefer older tissue. The first synthesis takes place when plants are only a few hours old; formation of ketones and alcohols follow after several days. Often, the biosynthesis of terpenes is subject to genetics and the changes in daylight.

Compounds with fifteen carbon atoms (sesquiterpenes)

Cis-6-trans-farnesyl-pyrophosphate is the biogenetic precursor of most cyclic and acyclic sesquiterpenes. Primary products are bisabolane, humulane, germacrane, and guaiane. The final structure of other sesquiterpenes is usually reached after several intermediates.

Triterpenes, cholesterol, sex hormones, steroids, heart glycosides

Two farnesylphosphate molecules form triterpenes with thirty carbon atoms from which cholesterol and consecutively via progesterone corticoid (steroids) and sexual hormones are formed. Other medicinally important products originating from cholesterol are heartglycosides (digitoxigenin) and vitamin D.

Molecules with twenty or more carbon atoms: diterpenes and carotinoids

Two geranylphosphate molecules form geranylgernanylphosphate, which is the precursor for most of the diterpenes (C20). Transformations in the plant lead to phytol, giberellines, steviosides, and aconite.

Decomposition products of carotene (C40)

Important plant odorants with very low odor thresholds such as ionone (violet and boronia), damascone (rose), and irone (orris) are decomposition products of Carotene.

Biosynthesis of phenylpropanoid components

Phenylpropanoids in essential oils are derivatives of the amino acid phenyl alanine, from which cinnamic acid is formed. Cinnamic acid is the precursor for anethole, methylchavicol, eugenol, methyleugenol, cinnamic aldehyde, coumarins, salicylic acid, methyl salicylate (wintergreen and birch), benzyl acetate (jasmine and ylang ylang), vanillin, piperonal (heliotrope), hydrochinones, and even alpha tocopherols.

Other processes

Some compounds of high odor impact, occurring only in low concentrations, are neither products of the terpene nor the phenylpropanoid pathways—they are synthesized along other routes in the plant such as along the lipid metabolism. Examples are aldehydes of high odor impact such as hexenal and nonenal, derived from linoleic acid. Jasmone, methyl jasmonate, and jasmine lactone are derivatives of linolenic acid

Complexity

Biological activity and symmetry

Essential oils are mixtures of natural substances that can be simple but more often range from the complex to the extremely complex. Commonly, essential oil components are subtly different from seemingly identical molecules that are synthesized. Often the natural original has different, usually better, activity than the synthetic counterparts. The usual reason is that essential oil components are pure enantiomes. Biological processes often will proceed with one enantiomer but not with the other. An example in which superior biological activity is tied to the biological occurring enantiomer is the oil of German chamomile. Only the natural oil with the enan-

Figure 11.1: Representative molecular skeletons of products of the mevalogenic acid pathway.

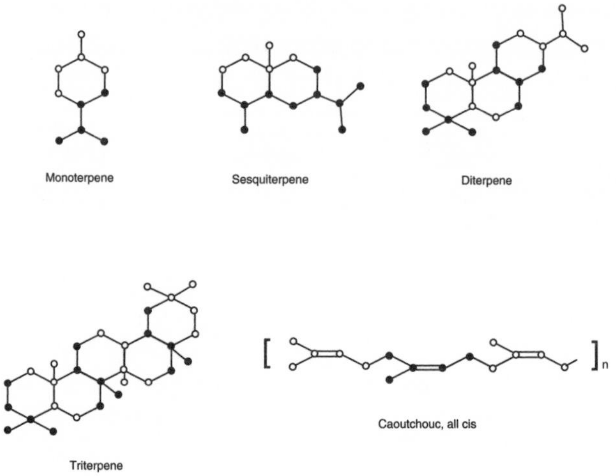

Monoterpene

Sesquiterpene

Diterpene

Triterpene

[ ]n

Caoutchouc, all cis

Black and white circles o •

denote how isoprene units bond together to form terpenes and higher homologues

Figure 11.2: Primary products of mono terpene synthesis.

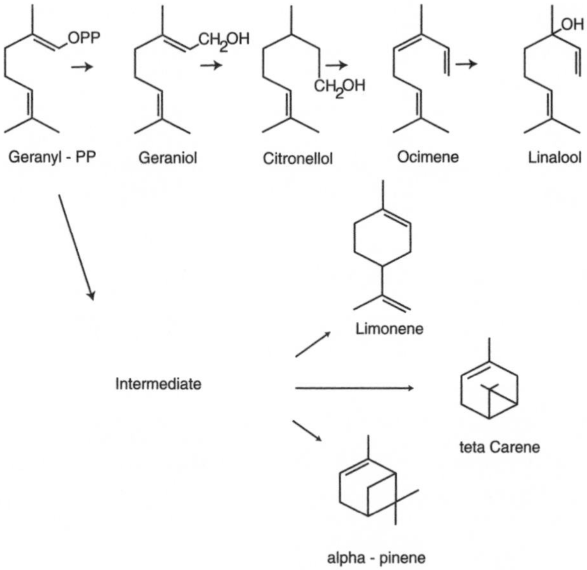

OPP → CH2OH → → CH2OH →→ OH

Geranyl - PP Geraniol Citronellol Ocimene Linalool

Limonene

Intermediate

teta Carene

alpha - pinene

Figure 11.3: Basic phenylpropanoids occurring in essential oils.

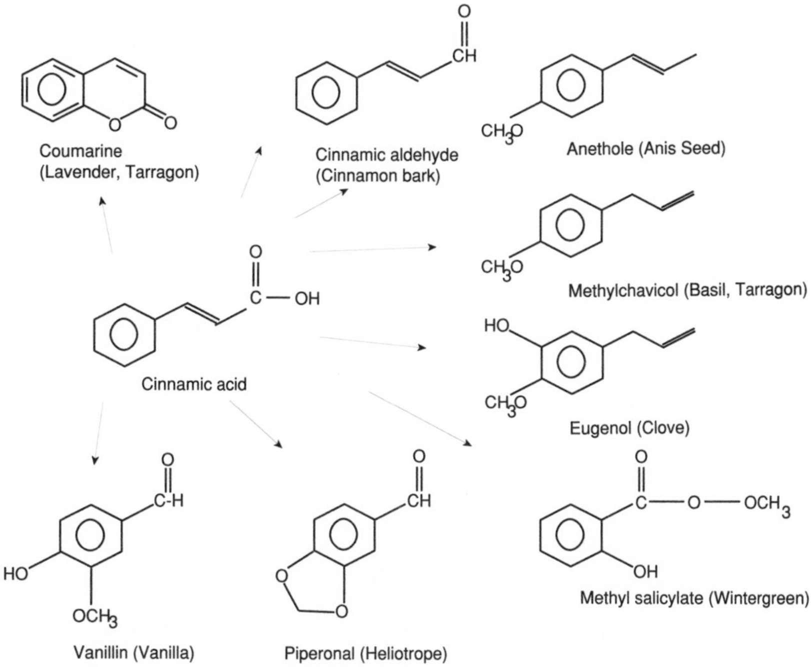

tiomerically pure (-) alpha bisabolol displays the truly impressive antiinflammative qualities. Synthetic bisabolol that is not enantiomerically pure but a racemic mixture of both enantiomers is distinctly less effective.
As the natural enantiomeric composition is often crucial for the biological effects of an essential oil, the topics of chirality and enatiomers shall be discussed in some detail below.

Chirality

Some of the most elegant features of essential-oil molecules depend on the symmetry of molecules. The most important type of symmetry is the plane of symmetry. An object is symmetrical if on passing a plane through the center of the object the reflection of one side of the object in that plane is identical with the other side. Such a plane is often called a mirror plane. If one half of the object mirrors the other half, the object is symmetrical. Objects exhibiting mirror planes include eggs, funnels, books, or a water molecule. An object without a plane of symmetry is asymmetric, such as trees and houses. A tetrahedral atom, such as carbon with all four chemical bonds being occupied by different entities, is asymmetric and such a carbon is called an asymmetric carbon. Right and left hands illustrate our recognition that two objects can be alike in every description except one—they are not mirror images of each other. They are not identical because they cannot be exactly superimposed on each other. In fact, for any object or molecule the ultimate test of asymmetry is to see if it can be superimposed on its mirror image. An asymmetric molecule can exist in either of two mirror image forms that are not identical. Such molecules with no identical mirror images are called enantiomers.

Optical activity

Differences between enantiomers exist but they can be detected only by devices that are themselves chiral, or asymmetric. Thus a pair of enantiomers will have identical melting points, boiling points, and so on, and will show identical reactivity towards most chemical regents. However, enantiomers show different reactivity toward other asymmetric compounds and will respond differently toward asymmetric physical disturbances.

The most common asymmetric tool is polarized light. If a beam of ordinary light is passed through a Niool prism, only part of the light emerges. The oscillating electric vector of the emerging beam is oriented in one plane the beam is polarized. If polarized light is passed through an asymmetric material, the plane of polarization is rotated, and this may be observed. Hence the asymmetric material is said to be optically active. The angle between the original and final planes of polarization is known as optical rotation. Measurement of the optical rotation of asymmetric compounds under carefully specified conditions provides a physical constant for characterization and identification of a substance.

Optical rotations of pure samples of enantiomers are equal in magnitude but opposite in sign. When the plane of polarization is rotated clockwise, the sign of rotation is taken as positive and the compound is said to be dextrorotatory (that is, rotated to the right). Levorotatory compounds rotate the plane of polarization to the left, or counterclockwise. The letters *d* and *l*, standing for dextro- and levo, refer to the sign of rotation. In the older literature the letters were often placed before the names of optically active compounds. Racemic mixtures are often referred to as *d l* pairs. Current practice is to use (+) and (-) signs to distinguish between enantiomers.

Manifestation in essential oils

Recently, enantio-selective analysis has become a powerful tool to ascertain the authenticity of essential oils. But these differences do not only give rise to a possibility for analysis, they are highly significant for the way these substances interact in nature. The pheromonal effects of terpenes, for instance, are extremely dependent on enantiomeric purity. This means, for example, that an insect will receive the message if a terpene is of the proper (+)

structure, whereas the other enantiomer or a mixture of the two will not be effective.

Impact on odor

The most tangible way to experience the differences between enantiomers of the same molecule, such as + and - limonene, is to smell the two isolated specimens. This has been done for almost any chiral odorant, and often very different fragrance impressions are observed. The interaction between an odorant of a specific symmetry and the receptor surface can be sharply different from that of the opposing symmetry. Following is a listing of some of the more familiar compounds that are found in essential oils, in either one enantiomeric form or another, and a description of their odor differences.

Extensive inventories of enantiomeric pairs encountered in known terpenes and sesquiterpenes in natural essential oils have been presented by Armin Mosandl and W. A. Koenig on various congresses recently.[3]

Table 11.2: Odor characteristics of separate enantiomers of selected natural odorants

Molecule	Odor Description	Oil
Linalool	R-(-) flowery-fresh, reminiscent of lily of the valley S-(+) differs slightly in odor	Lavender
(E)-Nerolidol	R-(-) pleasant, woody, warm, musky S-(+) slightly sweet, mild, soft, flowery, different from (Z), less intensive	
(Z)-Nerolidol	R-(-) intensive, flowery, sweet, fresh S-(+) woody, green like, fresh bark	Neroli

Limonene	R-(+) fresh, pleasant, orange like S-(-) faint mint note, turpentine note	Citrus peels *Mentha* sp., Conifers
α-Ionone	R-(+) fine violet like, fruity, flowery, raspberry like S-(-) strong woody aspects, raspberry like	Violet
α-Terpineol	R-(+) strong, flowery sweet, lilac S-(-) tarry, reminiscent of cold pipe	

Trace components

As analytical methods became more sensitive, researchers zeroed in on components present only in low concentrations. A driving force was the discrepancies in odor between reconstituted and natural oils. Known constituents of an essential oil are often mixed together in the proper concentrations, but the resulting reconstituted oil, even though it would yield a chromatogram practically identical to natural oil, would still have a markedly different fragrance. The conclusion is that there must be a small unknown fraction of hidden trace components with a very high odor intensity that contributes significantly to the fragrance of the essential oil. Jasmone and jasmonate compounds, with their green, celerylike odor, are important components of jasmine absolute, and damascenones, rose oxide, and similar compounds contribute significantly to the complete fragrance of rose oil. Recent research has discovered highly unusual molecules in essential oils with great odor intensity that often contain nitrogen or sulfur in addition to the expected carbon, hydrogen and oxygen.[4]

There is no relation between the concentration of a substance in an oil and its organoleptic value. Some compounds can be present in an oil in very high percentages and not imprint their odor characteristics in the essential oil strongly. Sometimes concentrations of a substance so low that it cannot be detected by gas chromatography can still be smelled. From the enormous odor impact it does not take a big stretch to imagine the potential therapeutic impact these compounds may have.

Table 11.3: Odor threshold

Values Of Selected Natural Products (ppb/water)	
Ethyl alcohol	100,000.00
Phenyl ethyl alcohol	1,000.00
Methyl eugenol	820.00
Beta-caryophyllene	64.00
Geranyl acetate	9.00
(+)-Nootkatone	1.00
2(E)-nonenal	0.10
Beta-ionone	0.007
Beta-damascenone	0.002
(+)-(R)-1-p-menthene-8-thiol	0.0002

While these trace components mostly contain either sulfur or nitrogen, the more common thymol or eugenol (made up solely of carbon, hydrogen and oxygen) can display the same behavior. The latter are the characteristic components in thyme and clove. In citrus oils such as mandarin, lemon, and orange, thymol and eugenol are present as traces and contribute distinctly to their odor.

The influence of trace components on the therapeutic effect of oils has not been evaluated sufficiently in aromatherapy. These components probably contribute significantly to the effect of an oil just as they do to their odor. In holistic aromatherapy the combined synergistic effect of all the components is needed to realize the full healing potential of a given oil.

Volatile nitrogen compounds

Almost every essential oil contains some nitrogen trace constituents compounds. More than twenty years ago, researchers detected a series of nitrogen compounds of high odor intensity in absinthe, angelica, carrot seed, coriander seed, clary sage, celery, galbanum, lavandin, parsley, petitgrain, rosemary, spike lavender, and vetiver.[5] Sulfur compounds also occur in almost every essential oil in concentrations from less than one part per *billion* to the parts per *million* range. The low concentrations in which these materials are present in essential oils do not allow their detection by normal gas chromatography. The most frequently occurring sulfur compounds are alkylthiols, dimethyl mono- & disulphides, dipropyl sulfide, diakyl thioesters, epithiocaryophyllene, and epithiohumulene.

White flowers such as jasmine, neroli, and hyacinth contain more nitrogen compounds, whereas red flowers such as roses seem to contain more sulfur compounds. In general, nitrogen compounds are found in oils from plant families Apiaceae, Labiatae, and Oliaceae, whereas sulfur compounds are found in the plant families Liliaceae (*Alium* species), Compositae, Asteraceae, and Rosaceae.

Safety of essential oils

Are natural substances generally safer than synthetics? The scientific viewpoint on this issue is summarized in the following quote:

> There is a growing trend toward the labeling of plant scents as "natural" with the implication that these are safe. (They may be better and are certainly more expensive, but this is not the subject of this chapter). The fallacy that "natural" is "safer" has been exploited in the food industry the world over, and is the principal foundation for the continuation of this belief among consumers.
>
> The fact is that there is no link between the natural origin of fragrances and their safety. All available data support the conclusion that fragrances made with natural ingredients are no more safe than those made from synthetic ingredients. Many synthetic fragrance materials are safer than naturals because of better quality control in their production and a resulting greater purity. To imply the con-

Table 11.4: High-odor nitrogen compounds in essential oils

Oil	**Odor descriptions of basic fraction**	**Identified Nitrogen Compounds**
Absinthe	strong green note, somewhat pealike	quinoline, alkylmethoxypyrazines (4)
Angelica seed	intensive green, pyrazine-like	akylmethoxypyrazines (4)
Carrot seed	green, pyrazine-like	alkylpyridines (6), alkylpyrazines (10), quinoline
Coriander seed	intensive green, pealike	alkylpyrazines (13), akylmethoxypyrazines (1)
Clary sage	strongly green, tobacco-like	alkylpyridines (2), quinolines (2), alkylmethoxypyrazine (4)
Celery seed	green bean, vegetable-note, rye bread connotation	2-alkylpyridines (2), alkylpyrazines (5)
Galbanum	intensive green, green bell pepper, galbanum-like	alkylmethoxypyrazines (11), tetramethylpyrazine
Lavandin	intensive note, fresh, green	alkylpyridines (5), alkylpyrazines (6), quinoline
Parsley	characteristic rye bread note	alkylpyridine (3), alkylpyrizines (9)
Petitgrain	strongly green, leafy	alkylpyridiens (6), azetylpyrazine, alkylmethoxypyrazines (3)
Rosemary	musty, leaflike	alkylpyridines (2), 2-acetylpyridin, alkylmethoxypyrazine
Spike lavender	green note	alkylarylpyridines (13), acetylpyridines (3), alkylpyrazines (7), quinoline

trary by aggressive labeling and advertising claims has no basis in fact and should be avoided by the fragrance industry.[6]

The published data on essential-oil safety assesses the safety of essential-oil components according to principles of objective science. Squeezing the substance of a vitalistic modality into the formalisms of official science may be useful to gain bureaucratic benefits such as state permissions, licenses, or transport insurance, but it does little to resolve the inherent question of whether or not natural substances are safe.

The tolerability of evolutionary substances has been discussed. To arrive at useful information in terms of safety, it is instructive to look at the abilities of plants to create toxic substances. Stinging nettle is fairly harmless, but only a little piece of a yew tree, or a few belladonna berries, can be deadly. Plants are not as helpless and defenseless as it may seem. They need protection because they are immobile. In their constant struggle for survival, plants have learned to recognize attacks and to guard against them. On the other hand, plants are the basis for most animal life, so herbivores come up with new methods to trick the defenses of the plants. This has led to a coevolutionary process over million of years between plants and their enemies. Both were forced to adapt to constantly changing conditions. Only gradually do researchers learn about the defensive strategies of plants, many of which are rather clever. The fact that plants form thorns is understandable. What is more surprising is that they are specialists of chemical warfare. Certain forms of potatoes develop proteins in the leaves that render the digestive system of larvae useless. Similar "appetite quenchers" are found in tomatoes and soybeans. Humans have known about these secondary plant components for a long time and some of them have been utilized for centuries: nicotine, caffeine, and phenols. The latter coagulate proteins and render them indigestible. Plum, apple, or almond pits protect themselves with highly toxic hydrocyanic acid. This fast-acting toxin is manufactured by more than eight hundred plant species. This prohibits the excessive feeding of animals on their seeds and therefore insures the survival of the plant species. Many of those secondary substances, in proper

Table 11.5: Essential oils and potential hazards

Oils	Potential problem
Citrus and needle	Can become an irritant over time, due to peroxidation. May be irritant to the skin, so careful testing on small patches of the skin, ideally inside the elbow, is warranted before the oils are used on larger areas.
Citrus oils	Should not be used on the skin before exposure to sunlight.
Peppermint oil	May cause shock in children under two and a half years, due to strong cooling sensation.
Clove and Cinnamon	Strong allergenic agents, (cinnamon bark, cinnamon leaf, *Cassia,* clove bud, and clove stem) provoke skin sensitization in approximately 5% of the population when applied topically. These oils are preferably used internally, which is less problematic.
Thyme, oregano, and savory	Skin irritants, used mainly internally.
Juniper and other oils with high terpene hydrocarbon concentration	May irritate and/or damage kidney tissue.

Oils with high ketone contents (Sage, Thuja, Wormwood, Hyssop) can be acutely neuro- and hepato-toxic.

dosage, have a long history of use in human medicine cabinets, such as atropin from the belladonna plant and digitoxin from foxglove.

The ability of plants to influence the hormonal balance of other organisms is not limited to toxins and poisons but includes the creation of an allure or symbiotic advantage for other species. This is most obvious in the very specific interactions between sesquiterpenes and human receptor sites, which are just being discovered.

The toxic substances in essential oils and plants are mostly well known to humanity. But nontoxic substances have interacted with the environment and organisms around them for millions of years and humans are well equipped to cooperate and coexist with them.

The possibility that scientists might be biased and the public right is shown by a recent development in Germany. Substances are often considered safe at first because the scientific methodology to ascertain their safety is crude and only takes into account quickly manifesting toxicity. Within the fast pace of commerce there is no room to assess the toxicity of a substance over a longer period of time. Polycyclic musk substitutes provide an example of so-called objective science doing little more than providing excuses for commerce at all costs.

These fragrance materials have until recently been hailed as safe and mass produced in staggering quantities. However, experts at various governmental watchdog agencies in Germany now see great cause for alarm: "The fragrance industry is increasingly producing synthetic musk substances for cosmetics and detergents which are even more problematic than their precursors, the notorious nitro musk compounds."[7] These nonindustry researchers are of the conviction that detailed studies for the potential toxicity of the so-called polycyclic musk compounds are urgently needed because the contact with these substances is practically unavoidable. These musk imitations are everywhere: in soaps, shampoos, body lotions, aftershaves, eau de colognes, detergents and fabric softeners, household cleaners, and air fresheners. Practically everything that is perfumed contains these substances. Now polycyclic musks are found in the fatty tissue of humans, in eggs and mussels, in mothers' milk and in fish. "Wherever we look, the concentrations of the polycyclic musks are drastically higher than those of the nitro musks. In certain situations 100 times higher."

These chemicals were patented in the 1950s and 1960s. At that time allergic skin reactions were the only hazard effectively checked for. Oral intake or the fact that the substances penetrate the skin was not anticipated. There are now reports that show that these polycyclic musks cause an increase in liver weight in mammals, often associated with tumor-promoting substances. The scientists cannot exclude the possibility that these polycyclic substances also belong to this class of tumor promoters.

The situation is typical. While the European Commission in Brussels is in the process of reassessing potential risks of the industrial musks, the industry points to dossiers that allegedly demonstrate the harmlessness of the two most-applied polycyclic substances, galaxolide and tonalide. The studies pointing to the harmlessness are basically industry-financed studies of RIFM in the United States. According to the data presented by the industry, consumers do not have to fear any negative effects and polycyclic musk substitutes do not have the potential for long-term effects.

Except there is one little catch. The dossier presented by the industry drew on unpublished private reports or personal communications to RIFM, not on published data!

Each person must decide where to place his or her trust: in the proven long-term tolerability of natural substances or the usual hide and seek played by industries when profits are on the line.

"Artisans have explored nature and its properties in order to learn to imitate her in all things, and to bring out the highest that is in her. Only in medicine has this been neglected, and therefore it has remained the crudest and clumsiest of all the arts."
—Paracelsus

TWELVE

Classifications of Essential Oils

An attempt to classify the components of essential oils according to their chemical composition was made as early as the understanding of organic chemistry permitted. A purely chemical approach led to the classification of essential oils according to the main functional groups encountered in monoterpene and phenylpropanoid molecules. Forty years later, Belaiche suggested classifying essential oils according to the functionality of their principle constituents. Franchomme and Pénoël, in their landmark work *L'aromathérapie éxactement*, continued this approach and attributed the pharmacology of essential oils to the pharmacology of their main chemical constituents. The compounds they wrote about reflect the tremendously broadened scope of chemical knowledge in the nineties. Following is a list of main types of molecules according to Franchomme and Pénoël:

Alcohols and phenols (hydroxyl group)
Phenol methyl-ether
Ether-oxides
Methoxycoumarins
Acetophenones
Hydroquinones
Ketones
Lactones
Coumarins
Phthalides
Aldehydes
Bi- or multifunctional compostions

Acids and esters

Acids
Terpenic and nonterpenic esters
Oxides

Hydrocarbon compounds (no oxygens)

Terpenes
Nitrogen compositions
Sulfur compounds

Pierre Franchomme also perfected and popularized experiments to assign what, for lack of better scientific terminology, must be termed "electric character" to essential oil molecules. The experi-

***Figure 12.1:** 'Structure Effect System' according to Franchomme and Pénoël*

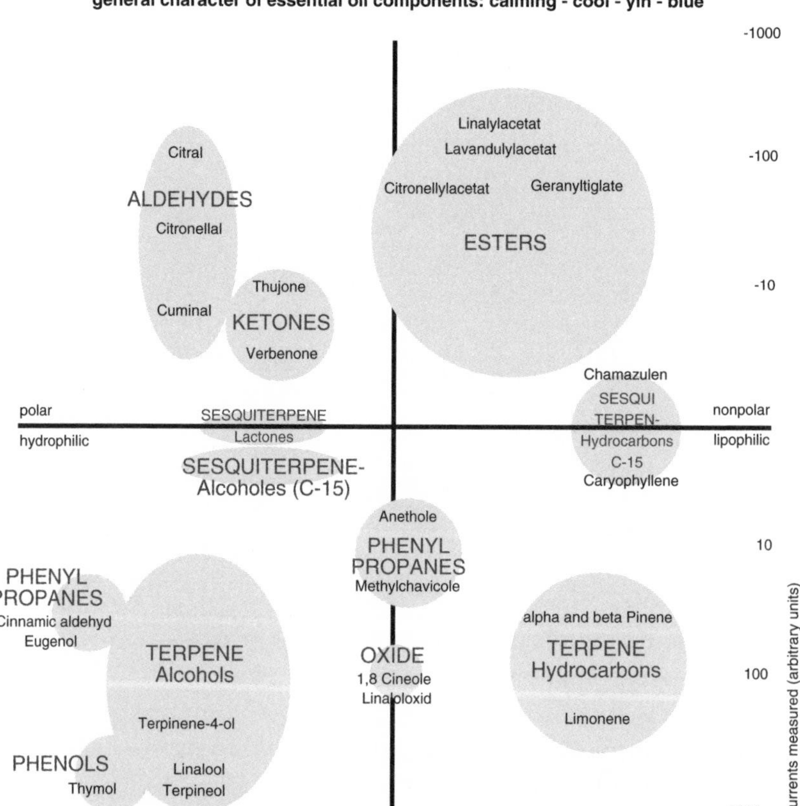

ment and its popularity within aromatherapy has done much to give the pharmacological classification of essential-oil molecules a sound basis. However, the experiment has not been repeated by other researchers, at least not as far as peer-reviewed scientific literature goes, and is therefore subject to critique.

A kaleidoscope of essential-oil components

The following constituents form the vast majority of all essential-oil matter (more than 99 percent) and provide all the main pharmacological effects—but not necessarily all the specialized effects that essential oils provide.[7]

Monoterpenoids

- *Monoterpene hydrocarbons:* Essential oils from citrus peels and needle trees (such as lemon, cypress, and *Pinus mugo*) have high proportions of monoterpene hydrocarbons. Monoterpene hydrocarbons have pronounced antiviral effects and exhibit a drying effect on the skin. Recently, antitumor activity has been described for limonene, a monoterpene hydrocarbon found in numerous essential oils. Needle oils are known for their decongestant effects in the respiratory tract.
- *Monoterpene Alcohols:* The monoterpene alcohols have strong antimicrobial effects. A unique combination of properties resembles, within the realm of aromatherapy, the effects of the tonic herbs of traditional Chinese medicine. Monoterpene alcohols, such as linalool (in coriander, lavender, and petitgrain), geraniol (in palmarosa), and citronellol (in geranium and rose), are well-tolerated and have some of the most appealing fragrances. The oils in which these alcohols are dominant may be used liberally and frequently and therefore have great value for maintaining balance, staying healthy, and preventing disease.
- *Phenol:* Thymol and carvacrol are forceful antibacterial agents. They are warming and strongly immunostimulant but can be irritant to skin and hepatotoxic.

- *Ester:* Monoterpenoid ester compounds have a distinct and rapid relaxing effect on the central nervous system and at the interface between the nervous system, the viscera, and the muscles. Esters relax, balance, loosen tension, and are spasmolytic. Oils with high proportions of ester components for instance Clary Sage, Lavender and Ylang-ylang, are well-tolerated and are suitable for liberal and frequent application.
- *Ketones:* Monoterpene ketones (examples are thujone, pinocamphone , and pulegone) display pronounced mucolytic (mucus liquefying) effects, especially in the respiratory and uro-genital tracts and on the skin. They effectively promote skin regeneration. Potentially acute neuro- and hepatotoxic effects. May be an abortifacient.
- *Aldehydes:* Monoterpene aldehydes (citral and cuminal) have strong antiviral effects, but they also display sedative and antiinflammative effects (citronellal and cuminal).
- *Cineole:* Cineole is the dominant compound in many oils from the Myrtaceae and Lauraceae families. Antiviral and expectorant properties are well known.

Sesquiterpenoids

- *Sesquiterpene hydrocarbons:* Sesquiterpene hydrocarbons can be powerful antiinflammative agents because of their ability to protect tissue by dissipating free radicals through conjugated π-electron systems.
- *Sesquiterpene alcohols and sesquiterpene ketones:* These compounds impart very specific effects that are unique to the given oil (vetiver, carrot seed, cedarwood, sandalwood, spikenard). Current research reports many highly specific interactions between receptor sites and sesquiterpenoids.
- *Sesquiterpene lactones:* Sesquiterpene lactones are, by far, the most powerful mucolytics within medical aromatherapy. They generally belong to most pharmacologically active principles found in essential oils.

Table 12.1: Representative Fragrances for 11 Main Functional Groups

The essential oils listed below have a fragrance that is essentially typical of the corresponding functional group and its characteristic compound.

Functional group	**Compound**	**Essential oil**
Aldehyde	citral	Litsea cubeba
Ester	tiglic acid esters	Roman Chamomile
Ketone	thujone	Sage
Sesquiterpene alcohol	cedrol	Cedarwood
Sesquiterpene hydrocarbon	mix of C-15 hydrocarbons	Gurjum balsam
Monoterpene alcohol	geraniol	Palmarosa
Phenylpropane (mild)	anethole	Anise seed
Phenylpropane (hot)	eugenol	Cinnamon leaf
Oxide	1,8-cineole	Eucalyptus polybractea
Monoterpene hydrocarbon	pinenes	Pine
Phenol	carvacrol	Oregano

Phenylpropanoids

- *Methyl chavicol:* The digestive, spasmolytic, and general antistress effects of this group of compounds is perfectly represented in basil, tarragon, and anise seed oils. They display a strong affinity to the autonomic nervous system.
- *Eugenol and cinnamic aldehyde:* Some of the most powerful agents in all of aromatherapy, these two compounds are highly antiseptic and have many different effects. They are suitable for rebalancing digestive flora.

The properties of a whole essential oil result from the limitless rearrangements and permutations that these eleven basic groups of constituents can undergo. Understanding the properties of the different essential-oil constituents has been beneficial to aromatherapy in the broadest sense. Reasonable pharmacological characterizations are more accessible for those users who need a scientific rationale for the applications of the oils.

Pierre Franchomme's structure energy chart and his entries for the various chemical families can be perceived as an assembly of little colored pieces of glass in a kaleidoscope. In it, one or all of the chemical families are constantly thrown into new arrangements, resulting in the composition of a new oil.

Certain sets of components occur repeatedly and are obviously preferred by the biosynthesis. Oils with a similar synergy smell alike and have similar pharmacological effects. The oil of lavender is a good example. Its two main components are the alcohol, linalool, and its ester, linalyl acetate. This synergy of monoterpene alcohols and their respective esters is encountered repeatedly, for instance, in the linalool type of thyme. The often-encountered synergy of alcohol and its ester combines the tonifying effects (of the alcohols) with the balancing and relaxing effects (of the esters). These oils are most useful for relaxing and stimulating day-to-day uses. A similarly important synergy is encountered in oils of the Myrtaceae family, which are distinguished by proportions of the terpene alcohols, terpineol (most often), cineole, and terpene hydrocarbons. Between these three types of compounds, the oils have very strong antiviral effects and are useful for upper-respiratory viral infections.

Essential oils generate physiological effects to which trace components often contribute dramatically. An example is cypress—its effects cannot be attributed to any of the main constituents. An evaluation of essential oils according to their dominant synergy is therefore a rather simplistic way to assess the more obvious pharmacological effects of these substances. However, the possible generalizations are still very useful. The finer or deeper effects of oils still have to be evaluated individually, which throws the modern aromatherapy user back to old fashioned empiricism—gaining knowledge experience by experience.

Figure 12.2: The Kaleidoscope Principle

cold

hot

a) all twelve basic families of essential oil components.

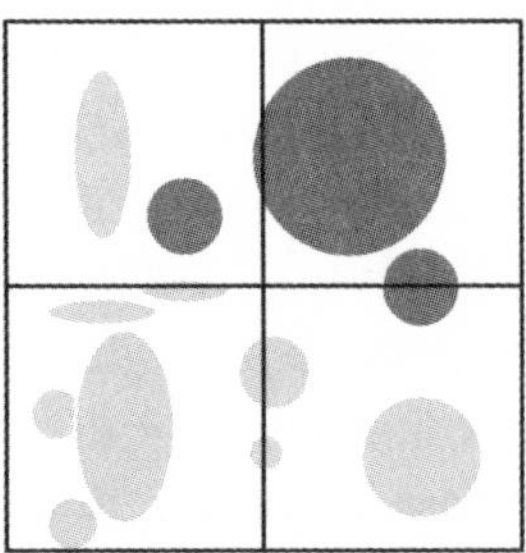

b) in Everlast the properties of sesquiterpene hydrocarbons, esters and ketones combine synergistically.

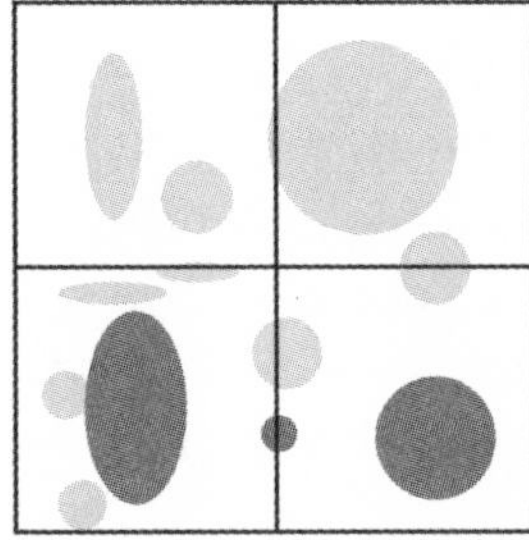

c) in Myrtaceae oils (Ravensara, Tea Tree, etc. the properties of terpene alcohol cineole and terpene hydrocarbons combine synergistically.

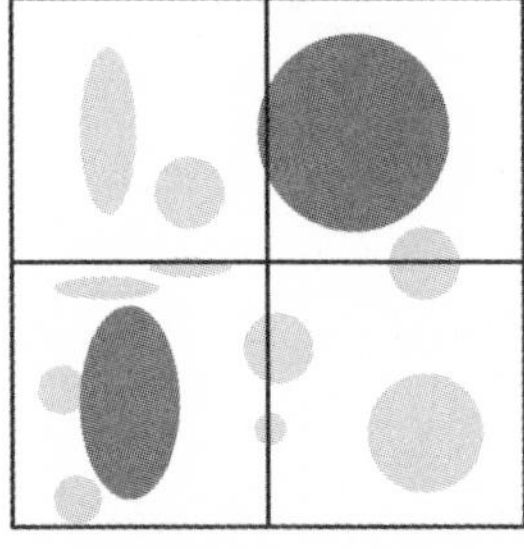

d) in Lavender the properties of terpent alcohols and esters combine synergistically

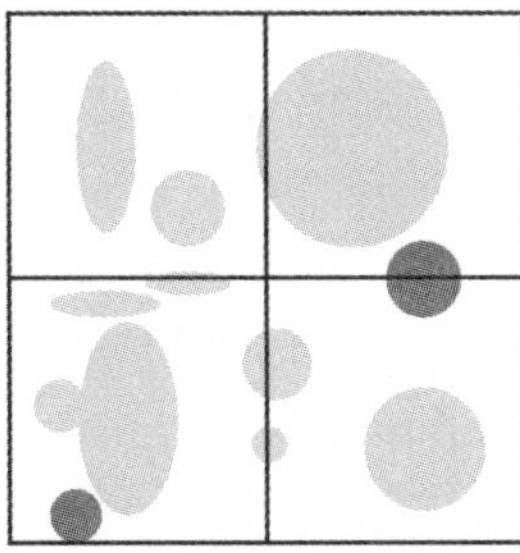

d) in Oregano the hot phenols are tempered by anti-inflammative sesquiterpene hydrocarbons.

Monoterpene hydrocarbon: citrus peel oils

Citrus-peel oils are composed of very high proportions of monoterpene hydrocarbons, particularly limonene (50–90 percent, depending on the oil), and a rich cocktail of trace components responsible for the complexity and depth of their fragrances. GC-MS analysis in the mid 1980s detected 143 compounds in bergamot oil, 153 in mandarin oil, and 93 in lemon oil. Of these compounds, approximately one half were discovered for the first time in these oils.[2] The characteristics of citrus-peel oils *(Rutaceae)* are determined by the monoterpene hydrocarbons but are distinguished by different influences from a broad range of larger molecules, such as the coumarins and furocoumarins, not found in other essential oils. The coumarin-type compounds found in citrus oils are too large to distill, yet since these peel oils are cold-pressed, these nonvolatile compounds are found in these oils. In addition, these compounds contribute to the photosensitizing action of citrus oils. As the fruits ripen, coumarin compounds decompose under the influence of UV light. Therefore, oils from late-harvested fruit contain fewer or none of these compounds. Red mandarin peel oil is normally free of photosensitizing coumarins for this reason.

Orange *(Citrus sinensis)*

The overall character of this essence is relaxing. It is particularly useful for anxiety and nervousness, and for these conditions it should be used as an uplifting and relaxing fragrance, either by itself or in combination with other similarly relaxing oils, such as mandarin or neroli, on an ongoing basis.

Preferred mode of use: Topical, fragrance
Caution: Photosensitizing.
Quality: Use organic only.

Grapefruit *(Citrus x paradisi)*

May contain up to 98 percent limonene. Grapefruit oil receives its olfactory character almost entirely from powerful trace components, one of which is the commercially isolated sesquiterpene nootkatone. Its pleasantly refreshing fragrance and rather affordable price makes it very useful for use in diffusers for disinfection of room air.

Caution: Photosensitizing.
Quality: Often dubious, use organic only.

Mandarin *(Citrus reticulata)*

True mandarin is distinguished from tangerine (from Florida) by the presence of small amounts of N-methylanthranilate, a nitrogen-containing ester, with pronounced relaxing qualities. This compound is not present in tangerine oils. Children almost universally like this oil, probably because its aroma might be reminiscent of sweets. It is a useful antispasmodic for cardiovascular, digestive, and respiratory systems. It soothes restlessness, especially in hyperactive children, and calms the activity of the sympathetic nervous system and ameliorates stubborn patterns of insomnia in combination with orange oil.

Preferred mode of use: Topical in massage, fragrance.
Quality: Ideally organic, although not much is offered in the world market.

Monoterpene/Aldehyde

Lemon *(Citrus limon)*

Recently, lemon-peel oil has received renewed public interest through the discovery of the antitumor effects of limonene. For use in aromatherapy, lemon oil should be obtained exclusively from organically grown fruits that are pesticide-free, because industrially cultivated citrus plantations are invariably sprayed with heavy doses of toxic chemicals.

Lemon oil has strong anti-infectious and antiviral activity. It can be used as component of blends aimed at liver regeneration and detoxification. Recently a range of influences of limonene on receptor-mediated processes has been documented, showing it to be preventative and curative for breast cancer in rats. Classic aromatherapy texts attribute fluidifying action on blood to lemon oil. Strengthens capillaries by diminishing their permeability.

Caution: Photosensitizing; potential skin irritant when peroxidized.
Preferred mode of use: Short-term only, internal or topical, do not use outdoors.
Quality: Use organic only.

Monoterpenes and the monoterpene/ester synergy

Monoterpene hydrocarbons were the first aromatic compounds to appear on a global scale. As these compounds developed in such abundance, the organisms containing them must have enjoyed distinct competitive advantages. These compounds represented an antiviral defense mechanism, which was critical for survival. Perhaps more interestingly, these compounds gave the plants an interface with the internal communication systems (receptors) of other organisms in a way that favored the emanating plant. We now know that monoterpene hydrocarbons interact with receptor systems, which originally developed in a hydrophilic environment, geared toward peptides. Botanical chemical engineering brilliantly overcame two obstacles: communication with the receptors of other organisms, and doing so with substances adapted to the stationary nature of plants by volatile substances that could travel through air: terpenes.

There are a number of needle oils that are used for their fresh fragrance and air-disinfectant qualities as well as for their decongestant effects on upper respiratory conditions. In both of these oils, the somewhat high-wired character of the monoterpene hydrocarbons is balanced by noticeable proportions of calming esters. Two specimens, *Pinus sylvestris* and *Picea mariana*, are distinguished from the bulk of the other needle oils by their hormone-mimicking effects. They contain hormone-mimicking, polycyclic terpenoid compounds. They are endocrine tonics, reestablishing hormonal balance in the pituitary, thyroid, adrenals, and ovaries.

Common or mountain pine *(Pinus sylvestris)*

While pine oil, like other needle oils, has varying anti-infectious and antifungal properties, its decongestant qualities for the upper respiratory tract dominate. It is a forceful tonic and adrenal stimulant. Specifically it can be used topically over the kidney area (10 percent in base oil) for adrenal support; adrenals produce, among others, adrenaline and prednisone, the body's natural cortisone.

Preferred mode of use: Topical only. Should not be taken orally.
Quality: Generally okay.

Black spruce *(Picea mariana)*

Individuals suffering from adrenal exhaustion may experiment with the essential oils of *Pinus sylvestris* and *Picea mariana* integrated with black currant absolute. A blend of these three may be rounded with other fragrances of individual appeal and can provide some very powerful synergies.

This may be even more effective as an adrenal stimulant than *Pinus sylvestris*.

Black spruce is a bronchial decongestant. It has a equilibrating influence on the endocrine system, which is especially useful for hyperthyroidism and adrenal depletion.

Preferred mode of use: Externally only.
Quality: Generally okay.

Bergamot *(Citrus aurantium* ssp. *bergamia)*

Most dominant in bergamot oil are its antidepressant and soothing qualities. It is useful for nervousness, agitation, and insomnia. It is anxiolytic and helps calm hyperactivity and anxiety.

Caution: Extremely photosensitizing.
Preferred mode of use: As fragrance or perfume.
Quality: Variable; many adulterated oils are on the market and identification of adulterated oils is not entirely trivial.

Monoterpene/Terpene alcohol/Cineole synergy

This synergy can appropriately be termed "the cold-and-flu synergy." It imparts a characteristic medicinal fragrance to these oils, which are associated with the expectorant action of chest rubs and winter baths. MQV (Niaouli), tea tree, *Eucalyptus radiata,* and other eucalyptus species all yield highly mobile, translucent oils of similar temperament. One of this group, ravensara aromatica, possesses a similar chemical composition yet, as a member of the dynamic *Lauraceae* genus, exhibits more uplifting effects.

Ravensara aromatica

Ravensara is of particular value because it is extremely well tolerated, whether inhaled or applied topically. Its mellowness is on a par with true lavender. Its tolerability and strong antiviral action make it the essence of choice for the treatment of influenza and shingles (together with *Calophyllum inophyllum*). It is a central-nervous-system tonic and its resulting uplifting qualities make it very useful during acute stages of the flu. May be helpful for insomnia (experiment with a blend of osmanthus absolute and ravensara).

Preferred mode of use: Internal, topical, diffusion.
Quality: Does not have significant uses outside of aromatherapy, therefore it's generally okay.

MQV or Niaouli oil *(Melaleuca quinquenervia viridiflora)*

Niaouli oil, or MQV as it is often referred to in aromatherapy, has a surprising variety of properties. Like many other Myrtaceae it is an excellent expectorant and also possesses moderate but distinctly useful antiallergic and antiasthmatic properties. It is an endocrine tonic with a special affinity to pituitary and ovarian glands. It strengthens and regenerates in cases of asthenia and has even been recommended to help alleviate arthrosis. When using MQV, it is best to experiment individually to establish a concentration that is well tolerated. To this end MQV is advantageously mixed with either tea tree, ravensara, and/or calophyllum to achieve a mix that is tolerated on the mucous membranes. You might start with a mix of 50 percent calophyllum, 25 percent ravensara, and 25 percent MQV. If this is easily tolerated, the MQV proportion can be made somewhat higher the next time the blend is created. Once a proper blend is established it can be used topically for hemorrhoids and genital herpes. It can also be tried for fibroids (with variable results). In French aroma medical practice, it is also used for hepatitis and dysplasias of the colon and to protect against burns from radiation treatment. It is a safe vaginal douche (mixed with tea tree).

Preferred mode of use: Topical.
Quality: Not many uses outside aromatherapy, therefore generally okay.

Tea tree *(Melaleuca alternifolia)*

Tea tree oil combines powerful antibacterial and antifungal action with an unsurpassed degree of tolerability. It is a virtual panacea or heal-all, yet its most important and reliable uses in aromatherapy are probably for bladder infection, candida overgrowth, and athlete's foot.

Preferred mode of use: Topical and internal.
Quality: Usually okay, but large-scale adulteration has also been reported!

Eucalyptus radiata

This is the most pleasantly fragrant of all eucalyptus oils; it is fresh with gentle citrus overtones. It has strong antibacterial, antiviral, and expectorant properties and is used in inhalations and topically for rhinitis, flu, otitis, sinusitis, and bronchitis. It's an excellent children's cold remedy in syrups, chest rubs, and vaporizers.

Preferred mode of use: Topical and inhalation.
Quality: Not many uses outside aromatherapy, therefore generally okay.

Monoterpene alcohols

Terpene alcohols are basically monoterpene structures with the addition of a hydroxyl (-OH) group. With the introduction of a hydroxyl group, the molecule gains an appreciable amount of polarity. Consequently, monoterpene alcohols are more hydrophilic than nonoxygenated monoterpenes. They are also less drying, less aggressive, and are much better tolerated by the kidneys than more lipophilic components. Because of their high tolerability, essential oils with high proportions of monoterpene alcohols may be used quite frequently, and with repeated use they can become very pronounced in their effects.

Recent research has confirmed that geraniol (palmarosa contains more than 70 percent), which is among the more commonly found monoterpene alcohols, has a superior ability to counteract pathogenic microorganisms and intestinal inflammation. The oil of *Thymus vulgaris*, thujanol type, is distinguished by a mix of monoterpene alcohols and has an impressive antimicrobial profile. Thyme thujanol is used in the treatment of chlamydia, salpingitis, and bartholinitis. This oil is as effective as the hotter, phenolic varieties of thyme, but is skin-friendly and generally much better tolerated.

Palmarosa *(Cymbopogon martinii)*

Palmarosa oil is distilled from a tropical grass and has a very appealing, roselike fragrance. It can be used with equal ease both internally and externally. It is nontoxic and nonproblematic, and is one of the most powerful, yet soft, antiviral oils. It also has very broad antibacterial and antifungal activity. It is useful for rhinitis, sinusitis, bronchitis, viral enteritis (intestinal flu), cystitis, vaginitis, cervicitis, acne, and eczema (dry and weeping). It is a uterine, neuro- and cardiotonic.

Preferred mode of use: Internal, topical, and as fragrance.
Quality: Inexpensive, therefore hopefully not adulterated.

Rose *(Rosa damascena)*

Contains up to 50 percent of the monoterpene alcohol citronellol. While the tonifying effects of the monoterpene alcohol are well known, the physical and emotional impact of a drop of rose at the right moment can extend far beyond those effects. If its medicinal and ritual uses throughout history are any indication, the amazing wealth of its diverse compounds never fail to interface with the psychosomatic network of man and woman.

Preferred mode of use: Perfume.
Quality: Only the true *Rosa damascena* from Bulgaria is convincingly sublime in every single year.

Thyme, thujanol type *(Thymus vulgaris thujanol)*

The essential oil of thyme, thujanol type, containing a variety of highly effective monoterpene alcohols (over 50 percent) is as much a product of nature as it is one of human interaction with nature. To maintain sufficient quantity of this chemotype for distillation, it must be cloned—propagated nonsexually—since the genetic disposition for its composition is recessive and would eventually disappear. Therefore, all plants of this chemotype that are collected for harvest have been cultivated by ongoing propagation through cloning.

This chemotype is a decidedly antiseptic oil equally well suited for external and internal use. In French aromamedicine it is formulated into a mild genital wash for chlamydia, cervicitis, vaginitis, and salpingitis. It's effective for influenza and asthenia.

Preferred mode of use: Internal, topical.
Quality: Only available from dedicated suppliers to the aromatherapy industry, therefore okay.

Coriander seed *(Coriandrum sativum)*

This oil is not extensively used in aromatherapy, maybe because of its varying quality. It is generally relaxing and antiseptic and especially beneficial for dyspepsia and conditions of the gastrointestinal tract. Because of its high linalool content, it can sometimes be succesfully used to replace rosewood.

Preferred mode of use: Internal.
Quality: Sulfur compounds may sometimes impart unpleasant top notes to this oil. Broad price range suggests that at least partial reconstitution is not unusual.

Alcohol/Ester synergy

Lavender *(Lavandula angustifolia, L. officinalis, or L. vera)*

Despite a big body of literature, both scientific and poetic, about the composition, uses, and the romance of lavender, there is precious little written on how to procure the *true* essential oil of lavender. Lavender hybrids, the *Lavandins*, are commonly distilled because they yield significantly higher volume. The total production of true lavender might average approximately twenty tons. And, easy as it is to calculate how many small vials that twenty tons can fill, what is routinely passed off as genuine and authentic *Lavandula angustifolia* is simply something else. The most reliable way to procure a true lavender oil is to purchase it from a supplier who can credibly assure the end-user that the oil originates from a clearly identifiable, even nameable source and has not been tampered with.

Thyme, linalool type *(Thymus vulgaris linalool)*

Nonirritant and effective systemic and topical anti-infectious agent, which is also highly suitable for skin infection and treatment of infants.

Preferred mode of use: Topical, suppository.
Quality: This is an aromatherapy specialty.

Geranium *(Pelargonium x asperum)*

There are many varieties of geranium oil, but the 'Bourbon' varietal has for years been considered the most desirable. Today, geranium oils from Madagascar are distinguished by the finest and fullest fragrance.

The oil is soothing and relaxing, ideal for massage and skin care. It has especially good antifungal properties.

Preferred mode of use: Topical, in massage oils and as a perfume.
Quality: Varies greatly.

Clary sage *(Salvia sclarea)*

A high content of spasmolytic linalyl acetate is one of the the dominant features of this species of *Salvia*. This is one of the most appealing antistress oils. It is a favorite for relaxing/euphoric massage and to assuage menstrual difficulties. It has been applied successfully for dysmenorrhea, oligomenorrhea, nervousness, spasmophilia, and nervous tensions. It is an effective yet mild antifungal agent.

Caution: May cause complications with conditions sensitive to estrogen
Preferred mode of use: Topical, as perfume, in massage.
Quality: Variable.

Neroli (*Citrus aurantium,* flowers)

This oil is a soothing and strengthening element in perfume compositions for exhausted nervous types. It facilitates birthing and eases post-partum depression. It is a hepatic and pancreatic stimulant. It contains the dimeric form of ocimene, a youth hormone, which might explain its effectiveness in preventing stretch marks.

Preferred mode of use: Topical and as perfume.
Quality: Sadly, importers are often unwilling to pay the real price for this oil. Clever marketing of cheaper substitutes is the norm.

Bergamot mint *(Mentha citrata)*

Not enough aromatherapy experience exists for this promising oil. Its tonifying qualities for nervous exhaustion are, however, well established. It strengthens weakened ovaries and is a male sexual tonic as well as a hepatic and pancreatic stimulant. It is especially effective for intestinal spasms.

Caution: Photosensitizing.
Preferred mode of use: Internal.
Quality: Generally okay.

Petitgrain (*Citrus aurantium,* leaves)

This oil combines an attractive price with a very pleasant fragrance. It has antispasmodic, sedative, and anxiolytic qualities. It calms the high-strung.

Preferred mode of use: Perfume, topical.
Quality: Variable.

Thyme, geraniol type *(Thymus vulgaris geraniol)*

This chemotype combines extreme tolerability with pronounced antibacterial and antiviral effectiveness. It works well for all upper respiratory and genital infections. Its characteristics should render it safe during pregnancy. Relieves intestinal distress caused by viral enteritis.

Preferred mode of use: Internal, suppository.
Quality: Aromatherapy specialty.

Terpene alcohol/Monoterpene synergy

Marjoram *(Origanum majorana)*

This oil combines antibacterial with spasmolytic properties. It is effective yet soft enough for children. Parasympathotonic. Best spasmolytic and antiseptic for whooping cough.

Caution: Not for asthmatics.
Preferred mode of use: Internal, one drop in syrup.
Quality: This oil is not produced on a large scale. If searched out carefully from genuine aromatherapy suppliers, it's normally okay.

Alcohol/Ester/Cineole synergy

Cardamom *(Elettaria cardamomum)*

This oil could use some more exposure in aromatherapy. It is nontoxic, gentle, and has an intriguing exotic fragrance. It has been shown to stimulate neurotransmitters, which induce its much appreciated stimulant effects on the digestive tract. A local anesthetic action explains the relaxant effects. It is also useful for strong intestinal cramps, the common cold, and bronchial ailments.

Preferred mode of use: Internal, topical, and as perfume.
Quality: So far no adulterations have surfaced.

Alcohol/Linalool oxide synergy

Hyssop *(Hyssop officinalis* ssp. *decumbens)*

It is important to clearly distinguish between the oil of *Hyssop officinalis* and the one described here, *Hyssop officinalis*, subspecies *de-*

cumbens. This oil is free of potentially toxic ketones, whereas the oil of *Hyssop officinalis* contains a high percentage of the ketone pinocamphone, which makes it one of the more potentially problematic essences to work with. *Hyssop decumbens* contains 50 percent linalool and 0.5 percent–1 percent (alpha & beta) linalool oxides. The oxides are responsible for the outstanding antiviral effects of this oil.

Sympathotonic. Useful for nervous depression, all upper-respiratory conditions, and asthma-related lung inflammation. Facilitates metabolic and liver secretions. Because of its mildness and strong antiviral properties, it is an excellent means for genital hygiene and prevention of STDs. After carefully establishing individual tolerance, the oil can usually be applied to healthy genital mucous membranes either undiluted or in a dilution of sesame oil.

Preferred mode of use: Internal, topical, suppository.
Quality: An aromatherapy specialty, but should only purchased from specialty suppliers.

Alcohol/Ketone synergy

Peppermint *(Mentha x piperita)*

This provides almost instant symptomatic relief from nausea and indigestion. Peppermint is maybe the most effective (among essential oils) stimulating liver tonic. Its analgesic properties have been demonstrated, especially for migraine headaches. According to published research, peppermint oil is liberally applied in a 15 percent dilution in rubbing alcohol to forehead, neck, and shoulders to treat migraine headaches. Its effectiveness in this application has been shown to be equivalent to that of conventional drugs. Peppermint is cooling and an anti-inflammative. It can open congested sinuses, relieve PMS symptoms, and help eye problems originating from the liver.

Spearmint *(Mentha x spicata)* and menthol are by far the largest items in the worldwide industrial aromatrades. As a result, the mints have received much attention in every respect: such as cultivation, the influences of breeding on the content of components, and adulteration. The composition and quality of mint varieties on the market vary widely and are victims of industrial standardization. Industrially produced peppermint in the sixty- to eighty-dollar price range is invariably steely and hard. Oils from small European distilleries are closer to the expression of the plant. Prices for such oils are distinctly higher but reflect the reality of genuine and authentic production practices. Interestingly, the genetic origin of aromatherapy's peppermint is not entirely clear. It is assumed to be a triple cross between *Mentha spicata, Mentha aquatica, Mentha longifolia,* and/or *Mentha suaveolens*. These varieties are also distilled simply by themselves and are available as essential oils in their own right. From an aromatherapy standpoint, they typically have very interesting compositions with applications for distinct conditions of the body.

Preferred mode of use: Internal in drop amounts or less and as trace to wake up otherwise unexciting essential-oil compositions.
Quality: Choose best possible; problematic oil exists as a result of industrial production.
Caution: Not for children under two and a half years.

***Eucalyptus polybractea,* cryptone type**

This oil was popularized by French researcher Pierre Franchomme and displays a unique pharmacology due to the presence of the ketone cryptone, in conjunction with other distinctive components.

The oil is recommended for conditions such as condylomas, uterine and genital warts, and viral dysplasia. Protocols with this oil prescribed in naturopathic clinics in North America showed variable success.

It is also a prostate decongestant and has antiparasitic and antimalarial (due to a content of australol) properties. Together with

MQV and sage, it has been recommended for endometriosis.

Preferred mode of use: Topically, in carefully established concentrations.
Quality: Available only from specialized suppliers.

Monoterpene ketone

Questions of safety in relation to ketone content in essential oils provide the world of aromatherapy with its own political issues. Ketone-rich oils have been shown to pose serious health hazards if ingested in excessive dosages (more than ten drops at a time for an adult). Acute neurotoxic or hepatotoxic symptoms may result. The exaggeration of these effects seems to have economic or political origins because the oils are highly beneficial, particularly as skin-regenerating agents. All ketone-containing essences should be used intelligently and in low concentrations by informed individuals.

Sage *(Salvia officinalis)*

Sage oil has been shown in vitro to have an extremely broad spectrum of action. Because of its high content of the problematic ketone thujone, experiences regarding this oil are gathered only slowly or not at all, despite the fact that published data support the conclusion that the whole oil is less toxic than the thujone content alone would suggest. Sage oil is highly regenerative. Because it dissolves lipids it is used against cellulite. It is antibacterial, antifungal, antiviral, and estrogen-mimicking.

Preferred mode of use: Topical in skin care, with caution in blends.
Quality: Variable.

Thuja *(Thuja occidentalis)*

Internal use of multiple drops of this oil is toxic. It is classically recommended for warts, yet its effectiveness, not unlike other wart remedies, is sketchy.

Caution: Abortive, neurotoxic.
Preferred mode of use: Externally only.
Quality: Variable.

Mugwort *(Artemisia herba alba)*

Internal use of this oil is toxic. As all its potential uses can also be performed with less toxic oils, it should not be used.

Caution: Abortive, neurotoxic.
Preferred mode of use: n/a
Quality: Variable.

Aldehyde

The characteristic tart, lemony fragrance of aldehydic essences (citral, citronellal) is exemplified in the oils of *Litsea cubeba* and *Citronella,* respectively. The one atypical exception is cumin, which contains the uncharacteristic cuminaldehyde. The citral-containing oils are strongly antiviral, whereas those with citronellal, *Citronella,* and *Eucalyptus citriodora,* are more antiinflammative and sedative.

Citronella from Ceylon *(Cymbopogon nardus)*

This oil is strongly antispasmodic and anti-inflammative; as it is rather inexpensive it offers itself to be integrated in compositions for frequent and liberal use. It has a moderate effect on relieving arthritis pain (used in a 5 percent solution in a base oil) and as an active and nontoxic component of insect repellents.

Preferred mode of use: Topical and in the diffuser.
Quality: Industrial product, variable.

Cumin *(Cuminum cyminum)*

In France this oil has been advanced as a perfect treatment for chronic viral diseases since its main aldehyde cuminal combines antiviral effects with (in such cases) much-needed sedative action. The use never really took hold, and it remains unclear whether this is due to its fragrance, which might be perceived as unfavorable. It is a good muscular spasmolytic and eases post-gastritis pain. It has a relaxing effect on the central nervous system.

Preferred mode of use: Internally.
Quality: Variable.

Eucalyptus citriodora

Inexpensive and relatively effective anti-inflammative for arthritis. (Works especially well when combined with *Helichrysum italicum*). Relieves muscular tensions. Its sedative qualities make it a useful candidate for the treatment of sleeplessness. This oil is often preferred over citronella since it has become available in organic quality from producers in East Africa.

Caution: Potential skin irritant.
Preferred mode of use: External.
Quality: Available in nonindustrial, organic quality.

Lemongrass *(Cymbopogon citratus)*

Like other oils with a high citral content, lemongrass can display valuable anti-inflammative and sedative effects. The trick is to use it in a concentration low enough to avoid any skin irritation. This is best achieved by blending it in small percentages with any number of other nonirritant oils such as lavender or rosemary verbenone. It balances the autonomic nervous system and acts as a vasodilator.

Caution: Skin irritant when unblended or undiluted.
Preferred mode of use: Internal, topical, and in diffuser, appropriately blended with other oils.
Quality: Despite being an industrial product, this oil is also available in a genuine and authentic quality for aromatherapy uses.

Lemon verbena *(Lippia citriodora)*

This oil parallels rose in its complexity. The clear effects of the antiviral and sedative citrals are complemented by one of the most impressive cocktails of high-impact secondary and trace components. The special quality of this oil is apparent in its gentle demeanor on the skin (caution: photosensitizing components are present!)—whereas other oils containing citrals are skin irritants, lemon verbena is much less so. Its activity and benefits for the endocrine system are unsurpassed. Precious and expensive, lemon verbena brings equilibrium and communication between all the major endocrine glands. Distinct endocrine activity.

Preferred mode of use: Internal, topical with caution because it's photosensitizing, and as perfume, by itself or in compositions.
Quality: Often extended or adulterated.

Litsea cubeba

See lemongrass for the necessity to dilute and/or blend. Used properly, it has anti-inflammative, calming, and sedative effects. It is an inexpensive substitute for the fragrance—not the complex action—of lemon verbena.

Preferred mode of use: Topical and in fragrance blends.
Quality: This oil is produced in China, and the quality available there is the *only* quality available. This means comparisons are almost impossible, yet the oil seems inexpensive enough to trust its unadulterated nature.

Melissa *(Melissa officinalis)*

True oil of melissa is for all practical purposes the most expensive essential oil on the market. Its yield is low and its distillation often difficult. It is highly effective on herpes lesions (but other less expensive oils also are). It is a powerful sedative; it prepares for sleep and ameliorates anger in crisis or trauma. It should be highly diluted to utilize its anti-inflammative properties.

Caution: Skin tolerance may vary.
Preferred mode of use: Internal, topical or as a fragrance, by itself and in compositions.
Quality: Available in genuine and authentic quality, but clever substitutes abound also.

Phenols

Essences with high proportions of phenolic compounds are as complex as other oils, yet they seem more one-dimensional because the aggressive, powerful, and stimulating characteristics of the phenols easily dominate the olfactory perception. This is typical for aromatherapy, where truly low concentrations are rarely explored. Using these oils in very high dilutions brings out their secondary effects.

Thyme, thymol type *(Thymus vulgaris thymol)*

Like all oils with a high phenol content, this oil has a broad anti-infectious spectrum of action especially good against pathogenic bacteria and yeasts. Lifts depressions caused by exhaustion and energizes.

Preferred mode of use: Internal.
Quality: Often industrial and variable, but genuine products are available.

Oregano *(Origanum compactum)*

Like thyme, this oil has a large spectrum of antibacterial, antifungal, and antiparasitic action and energizes during general asthenia. If anything, its effects might even be more forceful than those of thyme, albeit less complex. Oregano may not have the self-asserting influence on the thymus gland, which is alluded to in the name of thyme.

Preferred mode of use: Internally, ideally diluted in vegetable oil and in capsules.
Quality: Often industrial and variable, but genuine products are available.

Savory *(Satureja montana)*

A vaginal douche of a few drops of a blend of 1–2 percent savory with 98 percent tea tree oil stirred up homogenously in four ounces of water is recommended by Daniel Pénoël to treat vaginitis. This same blend can also be used in the morning, rubbed onto the body with a sponge, as a fortifying and immune-strenthening regimen to begin the day during times of increased risk of infection. Taken internally, it counteracts enteritis, enterocolitis, and nervous exhaustion.

Preferred mode of use: Internal.
Quality: Variable, but genuine products are available.

Phenol/Monoterpene alcohol synergy

Moroccan Thyme *(Thymus satureioides)*

Maybe the most effective for chronic infections and/or autoimmune diseases. It helps realign the immune system reducing chronic inflammation caused by pathologically elevated levels of gamma globulins. Aromamedicine uses this oil for angina and tuberculosis. Because of its highly restorative combination of carvacrol (a phenol) and borneol (a valuable terpene alcohol not encountered in similarly high concentrations in any other oil), it has also been recommended for arthrosis. Moreover, it is a sexual stimulant.

Preferred mode of use: Internal and external.
Quality: Produced only in Morocco. The available oils seem to be all of the same quality.

Ester

Roman chamomile *(Anthemis nobilis)*

While monoterpenoid esters are common in many essential oils, there is practically no other oil that reflects the nature of esters as exclusively as Roman chamomile. Despite its etherial fragrance, Roman chamomile has highly physical effects. It is a powerful antispasmodic and muscle relaxant that can be used as an emergency remedy during asthma attacks (rubbed on solar plexus, wrists, and temples) until more speciific help becomes available.

Preferred mode of use: Topical and in compositions.
Quality: Generally okay.

Sesquiterpenoids

Oxygenated sesquiterpenes and the sesquiterpene hydrocarbons have recently become a topic in receptor science. Receptor research advances on many different fronts, but a particularly fascinating area is the data collected on the constituents of medicinal plants used by indigenous peoples in the Amazon rain forest. Sesquiterpenoid compounds participate in active communication with a variety of receptor systems in the human body. They are known to have a wide range of biological influences, such as antineoplastic, antimalarial, antiviral, antimicrobial, and anti-inflammative effects.

These effects can be found in essential oils that contain a diverse group of sesquiterpenes paired with large proportions of monoterpene hydrocarbons, such as myrrh and frankincense, as well as oils that are almost exclusively composed of sesquiterpenoid components, such as vetiver. Due to the great complexity of these natural components, many unknown interactions between them and the various transmitter-receptor systems—with surprising implications for their pharmacological properties—can be expected to emerge with future research.

Sesquiterpenes/Oxygenated derivatives

Carrot seed *(Daucus carota)*

Small amounts of this oil (two drops per day) are used in convalescence to regenerate the liver. It is popular as a skin-care item, where it displays a distinct revitalizing effect on skin suffering from lack of tone.

Preferred mode of use: Internal and topical.
Quality: Fragrance and prices vary drastically as a result of differences in the production process and pronounced natural variation.

Cedarwood *(Cedrus atlantica)*

Cedarwood counteracts water and lipid retention and is therefore a staple in compositions against cellulite. It is a gentle yet powerful stimulant of the circulatory system.

Preferred mode of use: Topical.
Quality: Available from Morocco in what amounts to one standard quality. The oil is relatively inexpensive and should not invite adulteration.

Greenland moss *(Ledum groenlandicum)*

Highly specific and effective sesquiterpenoids make this oil the number-one choice for liver and kidney detoxification, especially after acute illness (taken internally, two drops per day). Aromamedicine recommends this oil for the treatments of nephritis. It is also quite effective in counteracting insomnia and allergies.

Preferred mode of use: Internally.
Quality: An aromatherapy specialty. It seems that adulterations of this oil have not been encountered so far, but it should only be purchased from trusted aromatherapy specialists.

Lantana *(Lantana camara)*

Called *cinco negritos* in Central America, this plant from the Verbenaceae family has very strong mucolytic powers and is used in the countries of its origin for chronic bronchitis and to ameliorate asthma as well as to treat varicose ulcers.

Caution: This oil could be neurotoxic and abortive.
Preferred mode of use: External.
Quality: Variable.

Myrrh *(Commiphora molmol)*

Myrrh corrects severe intestinal maladies such as dysentery. It is a poweful anti-inflammative, and despite its mild nature it has excellent antiviral properties. It deflates sexual overexcitation. Recently it has been found that sesquiterpenoid compounds found in myrrh bind to opioid receptors in the cerebral membranes and show structural similarity with opioid agonists. According to the authors of the study, receptor involvement explains the analgesic effects of myrrh and its widespread medicinal use throughout history.

Preferred mode of use: Internal and external.
Quality: Carbondioxid extracted oils offer assurance of quality. Steam distilled myrrh oil, when real, is quite expensive, and clever as well as primitive adulteration (with perfume extender diethyl phtalate) have been encountered repeatedly.

Frankincense *(Boswellia carterii)*

Frankincense can be successfully used for bronchitis and pain relief, for skin regeneration, antiaging wrinkle prevention, and to calm inflammative processes. Compounds in extracts of frankincense extracts have been shown to be uniquely effective against inflammative intestinal processes. Sadly, it is unclear whether the responsible compounds also occur in the essential oil. It could be that the substances in question are too polar and of too large a molecular size to appear in steam distillates—their presence would be more likely in CO_2 extracts.

Quality: Many commercial qualities are only remote derivatives of actual frankincense resin and remain therapeutically inert. But as expected, the beneficial effects are directly proportional to quality of distillate. Carbon dioxide extraction gives best assurance of quality. Products diluted with perfume extender are frequent.

Vitex or chaste tree *(Vitex agnus castus)*

The oil of vitex is a new and valuable addition to the arsenal of aromatherapy that has been distilled only recently. Previously, the herb was used exclusively as a tincture. Unlike any other oil, it actually improves progesterone levels, or more correctly it creates proper estrogen-progesterone balance in the second half of the monthly cycle and therefore eases or eliminates PMS. In fact, it alleviates PMS more effectively than all the other commonly suggested oils that mimic estrogen but do nothing to rectify the crucial balance between progesterone and estrogen.

Vitex has its effect not by supplementing or mimicking progesterone but by a distinct influence on the pituitary gland, which in turn generates proper equilibrium of estrogen and progesterone in the body. This well-known principle could not be attributed to a specific molecule in the tincture, and it is suspected that active substances are hidden among the oils over forty compounds that have not been identified.

Preferred mode of use: Extrapolating from the age-old use of the tincture, the oil is most likely nontoxic. Experimental internal use (one drop per day) has so far not resulted in any noticeable adverse effects, only great effectiveness in controlling PMS.
Quality: Available in genuine and authentic quality.

Spikenard *(Nardostachys jatamansi)*

Spikenard is probably the most powerful sedative in aromatherapy. It can be used universally in skin care, where it restores balance to all skin types. It can also be tried for otherwise difficult-to-treat skin conditions such as psoriasis.

Preferred mode of use: Internal and external. Blends well with lavender.
Quality: Spikenard of assured quality comes directly from Nepal. Other origins are more dubious.

Vetiver *(Vetiveria zizanioides)*

Vetiver oil is a powerful circulatory and immunostimulant. Receptor processes explaining vetiver's action on the circulatory system could recently be demonstrated in controlled experiments. Vetiver has a warm earthy fragrance that can strike an intimate chord with many individuals.

Preferred mode of use: Topical and in fragrance compositions.
Quality: The most reliable qualities seem to come from Central America.

Ginger *(Zingiber officinale)*

Ginger oil is as much a true tonic as the use of its root in traditional Chinese medicine would lead one to expect. It benefits most digestive problems and is immune-strengthening. Recent studies have confirmed ginger's pronounced effects on the digestive tract. In these studies, the pungent components of ginger were shown to inhibit cyclooxygenase and lipoxygenase enzyme activity in the arachidonic acid metabolic pathway and thereby reduce inflammation and relieve pain, as in rheumatic disorders and migraine headaches. Other compounds of ginger were shown to protect against gastric mucosal lesions.

Preferred mode of use: Internal.
Quality: Generally okay.

Patchouli *(Pogostemon cablin)*

Sadly, patchouli oil seems to be available mainly as an industrial product from Indonesia. The broad availability of inferior qualities seems to discourage a deeper exploration of the many beneficial properties true oils surely would have. The fragrance of patchouli oil improves with age.

Preferred mode of use: For fragrance use only.
Quality: Often disappointing.

Sesquiterpene hydrocarbon/Ester/Bisabolol structures

German chamomile *(Matricaria recutita)*

German chamomile oil is one of the most reliable anti-inflammative agents in aromatherapy. An overlooked quality is that it neutralizes toxic bacterial metabolic wastes, which are often the cause of fever during acute illnesses. German chamomile is an oil with distinct effects on the physical plane. It calms gastritis and stomach ulcers. To get the described benefits, care should be taken to utilize the (-) alpha bisabolol chemotype, which may contain up to 30 percent of this compound.

Preferred mode of use: External and internal for reliable qualities.
Quality: Oils on the market are often the less effective bisabolol oxide or bisabolon types, which contain little or no (-) alpha bisabolol. Depending on origin, German chamomile oils show great variations in price, pointing to the extensive industrial tampering to which much of this oil is sadly subjected.

Everlast *(Helichrysum italicum)*

Helichrysum oil has superior antihematoma and skin-regenerating activity. It regulates cholesterol and stimulates liver cells. It is a very good mucolytic and an effective free-radical scavenger, protecting newly formed cells.

Preferred mode of use: Topically, or internally in low dosages combined with lemon and rosemary verbenon to stimulate detoxification.
Quality: Available in genuine and authentic quality from dedicated aromatherapy suppliers.

Moroccan chamomile *(Tanacetum annuum)*

This oil has good antihistaminic and/or antiallergic properties. Can be used in blends for asthma (on solar plexus) and for emphysema (in diffuser: 10 parts *Pinus sylvestris,* 5 parts cypress, 1 part *Tanacetum*). Will calm down dermatitis inflammations resulting from many different causes. A very powerful anti-inflammative synergy for external use consists of 5 ml sesame oil, 3 drops everlast, and 2 drops *Tanacetum annuum.* This blend works as a first-aid remedy for painful sunburns or other situations where skin is actually damaged.

Preferred mode of use: External. It seems to display its strongest effects if its maximum concentration in a blend does not exceed 5 percent.
Quality: Available from Morocco. Even though some oils on the market work well for the described applications, some doubts remain as to the authenticity of the oil. The sweet, apple-like fragrance of more beautifully fragrant specimens of this oil was found to be due to synthetic fragrance materials in some cases.

Eriocephalus punctulatus

This oil is also a rather new entry to the aromatherapy arsenal. Its action, but not its fragrance, resembles spikenard or valerian. It is the aromatherapy remedy of choice for depressions and also for neuralgia.

Preferred mode of use: Internal and topical.
Quality: A specialty product, genuine oil is available.

Monoterpene hydrocarbon/Sesquiterpenoid/ Diterpenoids

Cypress *(Cupressus sempervirens)*

Essential oil of cypress derives its multiple uses from the action of complex sesqui and diterpene components. It is useful for all bronchial complaints and it is a choice spasmolytic for whooping cough. Aromamedicine recommends cypress for lung diseases like tuberculosis and pleurisy (in conjunction with *Myrtus communis*). It is a decongestant for prostate, veins, and the lymphatic system. Its bitter principles strengthen a weak pancreas. It is an intestinal and neurotonic. It helps to prevent the spread of varicose veins, hemorrhoids, and edema, especially of the lower limbs.

Preferred mode of use: Internal and topical.
Quality: Often uncertain.

Monoterpene hydrocarbon/Sesquiterpene hydrocarbon/Aliphatic hydrocarbons

St. Johnswort *(Hypericum perforatum)*

The essential oil of St. Johnswort is as gentle as the lore of the plant would indicate. Aromamedicine recommends it for counteracting kidney infections and trauma. The oil is deeply penetrating and more volatile than other essential oils. It is precious and rare.

Preferred mode of use: Internal and external.
Quality: As an aromatherapy specialty, generally okay.

Phenylpropanoid molecules

Phenylpropanoid compounds were among the first ones to be isolated and synthetically produced in the nineteenth century. The basic structure shared by all compounds in the phenylpropanoid group is the aromatic phenyl ring with a 3-carbon or propene side-chain. This structure is derived from the amino acid phenylalanine, and is present in essential oils in many variations—all of which are physiologically highly active.

An empirical classification of phenylpropanoids occurring in essential oils recognizes their most immediate and tangible qualitites—hot or mild. Hot phenylpropanoids are defined as those most likely to cause dermatitis and skin irritation (eugenol or cinnamic aldehyde). Mild phenylpropanoids are those that are gentle—among others, the phenylpropene ethers anethole and estragole.

Phenylpropanoids are the dominant products of the secondary plant metabolism at the beginning of the development of angiosperms. As this development progressed to more highly organized angiosperms, products of the mevalonic acid pathway (terpenes) became prevalent in angiosperms. Today, eugenol, the main constituent of clove oil, and cinnamic aldehyde, the main constituent of cinnamon bark oil, are among the most thoroughly researched components of essential oils. Within modern times, the move toward commercialization has made these two oils almost outcasts in the litmus test of aromatherapy. This may also be a reflection of the predominant use of aromatherapy for massage in Great Britain and the limited usefulness of these oils for topical applications, because they do pose hazards such as dermatitis reactions to those with sensitive skin. Nonetheless, their ability to restore equilibrium to the intestinal flora, to act against pathogens, and to be metabolized by the good bacteria makes them indispensable agents in maintaining balance during an illness. Another reason that these oils are so highly contested may rest in their extreme effectiveness. In casual aromatherapy, it is customary to always use at least a drop or two. Doing so with cinnamon or clove results in too high a concentration.

A more accurate evaluation of the qualities of these two oils is given by Dr. Deininger, of Cologne, Germany, who put it this way:

"If people in the world knew about all the beneficial properties of cinnamon it would not be available anymore, it would be soaked up from the market in no time."

One convenient and uncomplicated way to feel the power of eugenol is to use bay laurel oil. This oil contains approximately 15–30 percent eugenol within a diverse mix of monoterpene alcohols and esters and a small amount of phenylpropane ethers, cineole, and sesquiterpene lactones. This creates a natural balance, a matrix, in which the eugenol is suspended and does not have the same fierce reactions on the skin as it would if it were isolated or in the form of clove oil where it is present in a much higher concentration.

The softer phenylpropanoid ethers (anethole and estragole) found in tarragon, basil, and anise seed, when tested as isolated substances, were not as effective against microorganisms as eugenol and cinnamic aldehyde isolates. However, recent studies demonstrated that oxidation products, which occur in the body when these compounds are metabolized, do in fact exhibit very powerful antimicrobial effects. Eugenol showed pronounced antimicrobial effect against all gram(-) and gram (+) microorganisms tested.

Phenylpropane ether

Anise seed *(Pimpinella anisum)*

A drop of anise seed oil on a sugar cube will immediately restore equilibrium to an acutely out-of-whack autonomic nervous system. It is the number-one hangover remedy. It has an estrogen-mimicking effect and can be used for amenorrhea.

Preferred mode of use: Internal.
Quality: Generally okay.

Phenylpropane ether/Coumarin synergy

Tarragon *(Artemisia dracunculus)*

Tarragon oil is a powerful intestinal, neuromuscular, and female reproductive system spasmolytic. Aromamedicine recommends it for hepatitis A and B. It has antiallergic properties and calms in cases of colitis. Tarragon oil can also be used as a first-aid remedy for shock, until professional help becomes available.

Preferred mode of use: Internal.
Quality: Generally okay.

Eugenol/Terpenoid ester/Cineole synergy

Bay laurel *(Laurus nobilis)*

Bay laurel is one of the most effective all-round strengthening and preventive oils. It has superior expectorant, mucolytic, viricide, and antifungal properties. It is effective against candida (albicans, tropicalis and pseudo-tropicalis) and a broad range of pathogenic bacteria, including staphylococcus, streptococcus, enterococci, gonococci, pneumococci, E. coli, and klebsiella. It is much milder than clove oil and can be used more liberally.

Preferred mode of use: Internal and topical.
Quality: Oils from the northern Mediterranean have a lower cineole content and a much more appealing fragrance than those from North Africa.

Basil *(Ocimum basilicum)*

Oils distilled from cultivars of basil from different global bioregions are some of the most varied encountered among all essential-oil plants. Basil exemplifies the degree of flexibility and ability to adapt that the more highly evolved angiosperms have mastered. Traditionally, basil oil has been recommended as a cerebral stimulant. For a brief listing of major cultivars and properties, see the charts on page 33.

Preferred mode of use: Internal and topical and in fragrance compositions.
Quality: Ranges from industrial to exquisite.

Cinnamic aldehyde

Cinnamon *(Cinnamomum zeylanicum)*

According to the work of Deininger as well as Franchomme and Pénoël, cinnamon bark oil is effective against 98 percent of all pathogenic gram (+) and gram (-) bacteria. It is also effective against yeasts, candida (albicans, tropical, pseudo-tropical) and fungi, including aspergillus, thereby preventing aflatoxin production. It is antiparasitic and prevents fermentation in the intestines; it is effective against diarrhea, colitis, amoebic dysentery, enterotoximia, bacterial cystitis, and urinary tract infections with E. coli and tropical infections accompanied by fever.

Caution: potential skin irritant and sensitizing agent.
Preferred mode of use: Internally.
Quality: Genuine qualities are available but adulteration is also common.

Eugenol (containing a free phenolic hydroxyl)

Clove bud *(Eugenia caryophyllata)*

Contains up to 70 percent eugenol, 22 percent esters, and 5 percent sesquiterpenes. It has antiviral and antifungal effects. Essential oil of clove has an impressive range of action against pathogens and illnesses of all kinds. It is antiparasitic and works for gum infections, toothaches, and tonsillitis. Research indicates its usefulness for poliomyletis, multiple sclerosis, tuberculosis, cholera, Hodgkins disease, hepatitis, malaria, viral colitis, dysentery, amoebas, spasmodic colitis, thyroid imbalance, arthritis, viral neuritis, neuralgia, salpingitis, and cystitis.

Caution: Potential skin irritant and sensitizing agent.
Preferred mode of use: Internal use only unless highly diluted.
Quality: Generally okay.

Phenylpropanoid derivatives

Precursors to phenylpropanoid structures encompass a very wide range of compounds that are, in correct chemical terminology, not phenylpropanes but derivatives of benzoic or phenylacetic acid. The origin of typical esters found in ylang ylang, jasmine (benzyl acetate), wintergreen (methyl salicylate), sassafras (benzyl salicylate), and the typical aldehydes found in heliotrope (piperonal) and vanilla (vanillin) are present on the biosynthetic pathway starting with phenylalanine and cinnamic acid.

Ylang ylang *(Cananga odorata)*

At least three different fractions of ylang ylang oil are collected during distillation: the earliest, the lightest and most ethereal fragrance, and the one collected during the last hours of the distillation, which is thicker and smokier than the earlier ones. True ylang ylang is distilled from *Cananga odorata genuina,* whereas a somewhat lesser oil is distilled from *Cananga odorata macrophylla,* the latter refered to as *Cananga* oil. Ylang ylang impresses with its sublimely sweet and narcotic fragrance. It is a powerful antispasmodic and calms tachycardia and hypertension. While the oil itself is probably not a stimulant, the allure of its fragrance give it aphrodisiac overtones.

Preferred mode of use: Topical and in fragrant blends.
Quality: Quite variable.

Wintergreen *(Gaultheria fragrantissima)*

For a long time, wintergreen oil was really synthetic salycilate. But for a number of years now, true distilled oil is again available from Nepal, distilled not from *Gaultheria procumbens,* as in North America, but from *Gaultheria fragrantissima*. The oil is traditionally used for its anti-inflammative and analgesic effect—mediated by a process known as counterirritation—for rheumatoid arthritis. The oil is highly irritant if used in too high a concentration. It should always be blended with other essential oils.

Caution: Skin irritant use in high dilutions.
Preferred mode of use: External.
Quality: Either genuine or synthetic.

"But where there is danger, a remedy also grows."
—Friedrich Hölderlin

THIRTEEN

Applications

Because essential oils can be used medicinally, the adopted mode of application often reflects conditioning received from the medical system. We tend to apply oils in the same fashion conventional medicines are applied, for example, three drops three times a day, simply because it is our learned behavior from doctors' prescriptions. This form of application is not harmonious with the nature of the oil but subconsciously reinforces the conditioning of the conventional medical system. To allow aromatherapy to work as well as possible, application methods should be chosen that are consistent with the nature of the oils, such as the fact that they are liquid, lipophilic, aromatic, volatile, and made up of very small molecules.

Due to their physical properties, essential oils make the way they are administered somewhat less crucial. This means that often more than one way of application can be correct; there is ample room for personal preference. However, excessive dosages need to be avoided.

Conventional medicines normally work by entering the metabolism via the stomach, small intestine, and liver. The molecules in the medicines have no other way to enter the body. Essential oils are made up of very small lipophilic and volatile molecules. This gives them much greater overall mobility into and within the body, especially skin and fatty tissue. They are aromatic, which gives them the ability to influence behavior. Essential oils are different in their physical properties from most conventional drugs and should be applied in a way that utilizes these different physical properties. Topical application and inhalation are often very effective.

Diluting oils

The most common way to transfer essential oils from the bottle onto the skin is to dilute them in a fatty-base oil and to use the mixture as an ointment or massage oil. Extensive literature exists, especially in the skin-care industry, on the pros and cons of various fatty oils. Different individual preferences may exist, but certain criteria have evolved over time. Almond oil is a well tolerated, light, nonintrusive base oil for massages with a faint or no fragrance. Hazelnut generally contains small percentages of desirable polyunsaturated fats and vitamin E. For the treatment of inflammatory conditions, sesame oil holds an advantage over other oils because it contains small concentrations of free-radical-quenching triterpenoids that form effective synergies with antiinflammative essential oils. The quality of the vegetable oil is very important; organic quality helps to avoid unwanted skin reactions.

A 2 percent dilution of essential oil in a base oil has emerged as the standard suggestion for skin care and massage oils. For specific therapeutic applications, concentrations higher than 2 percent are sometimes suggested. A concentration of 10 percent of essential oils in a base oil has a feel quite close to an undiluted oil. But concentrations below 2 percent have also proven effective, particularly in skin care, when the essential oils used are exclusively genuine and authentic.

Table 13.1: Intrinsic properties of essential oils

Property	Oils	Pills
Molecular size	small	medium to large
Solubility	in fatty oils	mostly in water
Composition	often complex, hundreds of different molecules	Single substance or mixture of few substances
Origin	plant biosynthesis	mostly synthetic from chemical factory
Mode of action	multilayered and cooperative. Similar possibilities as pills but also many more holistic influences on hormone balance and the autonomic nervous system. Odor effects, on emotions and psyche. Oils support healthy processes (cooperative).	Pharmacological: provable effects are the main feature. Side effects are often tolerated but undesirable and potentially risky. Pills work mainly antagonistically, fighting microorganisms or symptoms

Table 13.2: Applying oils consistent with their nature

Aspect of the oil	Application consistent with specific aspect
Fluid	With other fluid, such as water, in the shower or bath. or fatty oils via carrier oils
Volatile	Inhalation or room fragrancing.
Aromatic	As perfume with olfactory, psychological, and hormonal effects.
Lipophilic	Topical for skin care and massage, utilizing their pentrating power

Undiluted oils

Sweeping generalizations—such as not using undiluted essential oils at all on the skin—do not do justice to the complexity of aromatherapy. There are scenarios in which an essential oil in a 2 percent dilution in a base oil could still create considerable skin sensitization and discomfort, and there are other scenarios in which the undiluted application of an essential oil is perfectly reasonable and beneficial. Undesirable effects usually are the consequence of using industrial and adulterated oils and not the consequence of the wrong concentration. Nonetheless, certain oils are frequently known to cause skin sensitization and therefore need to be used with the appropriate cautionary methods (for essential oils and skin sensitization see page 174.

The lipophilic nature of essential oils makes for unique applications in conjunction with water, such as in a bath or in a shower. Oils and water, of course, do not mix. Essential oils, however, do mix readily with lipophilic environments. Skin tissue is, at least compared to water, a lipophilic environment. Essential oils applied to the skin in the bath or in the shower will have an increased tendency to dissolve in or penetrate the tissue rather than remain in the water. Interrupting your shower for a short time will allow the essential oils to reach their full effect on your skin. The beneficial stimulating or relaxing effects essential oils can have in the bath are sufficiently explored in the literature.

Inhalation

Inhalation of the appropriate essential-oil mixtures can be very effective for containing oncoming colds or bronchitis conditions. One of the best methods is to use the empty plastic shell of a typical asthma inhaler filled with tissue with a drop of essential oil on it. Another effective way to inhale essential oils is to put one or two drops on a two-inch-by-two-inch piece of paper tissue, rolling the paper and placing it gently it into the nostrils.

Diffusers and aroma lamps have been a staple of the aromatherapy-products industry for a while and are found in many homes. Diffusing essential oils in this fashion has far-reaching benefits, such as drastically reducing microorganisms in room air. This is especially useful when sick family members are taken care of in the house. Diffusing essential oils in rooms and buildings is also an effective method of keeping fungal infestations away and reducing the spore count. The diffuser utilizes a jet stream of air to disperse oils and does not subject them to temperature. Because no temperature strain is placed on the oil, it is dispersed in its complete form. Aroma lamps use heat to evaporate the oil—lighter components will evaporate more quickly and the less volatile components often remain in the dish.

Internal application

While the application of essential oils via the skin is often the most effective form of treatment, there *are* instances in which using essential oils internally is appropriate. Again, their unique fluid and lipophilic nature has to be taken into account. In order to deliver essential oils successfully to the stomach and/or the small intestines, they must be absorbed into an appropriate carrier material or be emulsified in liquid. One or two drops will deliver the full pharmacological effect that can be gained from any given oil. Ingesting essential oils in their natural state will result in a fair degree of absorption in the mouth and esophagus; only a little oil will actually reach the stomach.

French medical aromatherapy commonly applies essential oils via suppositories. Concentration levels for adults are typically 10 percent essential oil in a suppository mass. This is 7–8 drops; or a total of 300 mg per 3 g suppository as the upper limit. For children, a total of 1 drop or 25 mg per 1 g suppository is appropriate. Applying essential oils rectally is especially advantageous for the treatment of lower respiratory conditions. By being absorbed into the rectal veins, essential oils bypass the liver and reach the heart-lung circulatory system, the lower bronchial tract, and the other organs without having been altered by the liver metabolism.

How to approach self-help responsibly

Though excessive use of oils can irritate the skin, such unpleasant experiences are generally only temporary. What generally happens is that too much use of the same undiluted oil may eventually cause sensitivity to this oil, regardless of how gentle or soft the oil really is. However, no permanent harm will come from making a mistake once or twice and enduring some unpleasant but brief effects from certain oils. This is part of aromatherapy, part of learning and gaining a better understanding of the self-medication process, which will enrich our experiences and enable us to trust, when we apply oils again, that small amounts are able to do the job. Trust replaces the "more is better" conditioning that is implicit in most other consumer products.

In choosing aromatherapy, the layperson is on his or her own. This can be disconcerting, but does not take away from the potential for success. To attempt self-healing is an entirely new experience for many. When working and gathering experiences with essential oils, one must expect the unexpected and constantly raise questions. The safety of aromatherapy allows for experiences both pleasant and unpleasant, both useful and useless, making it effective among family and friends who share and exchange information. It is for those who have true healing in mind. Nonetheless, some essential oils need to be used with the appropriate caution.

The logic for treating conditions is simple: don't choose conventional medicine where aromatherapy will do, and use aromatherapy within its therapeutic parameters. Aromatherapy should be used for conditions that allow it to work safely and easily. Aromatherapy also is an excellent starting point to explore other alternative methods of healing.

Allopathic medicine should be chosen for what it does best:
- trauma management
- diagnosis and treatment of surgical emergencies
- prevention of some infectious diseases by immunization
- replacement of hips, knees, and other damaged body parts
- reconstructive surgery
- diagnosis of hormonal deficiencies

Alternatives should be chosen where allopathic medicine fails:
- treatment of viral infections
- cures for most chronic degenerative diseases
- effective management of many kinds of mental illness
- most forms of allergy or autoimmune diseases
- management of psychosomatic illnesses
- cures for most forms of cancer

Aromatherapy works *best* for:
- infections and acute conditions especially susceptible to quick intervention
- improving immune response

Aromatherapy works *well* for:
- nervous-system imbalances
- psychological and hormonal imbalances

Aromatherapy works *fairly well* for:
- autoimmune diseases. (These conditions are often the result of many years of assault on the body that led to seriously impaired or permanently destroyed body functions.)

While it is possible to achieve specific goals, aromatherapy supports a return to a state of improved unity of body and mind. Essential-oil therapy rids the body of toxins instead of suppressing reactions to them, returning the body to a healthier state than before the onset of the disease. Individuals who have always relied on allopathic medicine and have manifested diseases cannot simply switch over to a new healing paradigm. Established patterns are deeply ingrained and it is unwise and irresponsible to force too much of a change. Still, these individuals can often be helped if they use oils to stimulate metabolic function.

Upper respiratory conditions

The holistic view of colds, which considers all metabolic processes involved, is the basis for designing treatment strategies that are much more effective than simply "shooting" at germs. The principle of germs as a cause for colds is highly overestimated. While the germs credited with causing colds are present at all times, not everyone contracts a cold at the same time; a cold takes hold when the body is weakened and the immune response is low. Infection processes like the common cold really are the consequence of a temporary immune depression. Regular use of immunostimulant essential oils effectively prevents colds or at least diminishes the strength of their symptoms. Aromatherapy should be complemented with traditional Chinese medicine, because its herbal remedies are extremely effective.

If aromatherapy is implemented when the symptoms are already fully developed, a cold will not be averted. Still, therapy with essential oils will cause a faster disappearance of the symptoms and minimize unpleasant accompanying effects. Recurrence is discouraged or avoided by improving the immune response.

Contracting and overcoming a cold is connected to the immune functions of the respiratory tract. In the nasal cavities, air is moistened and cleaned. The mucous membranes establish a constant temperature inside the nose of approximately 88–93 degrees. Immunocompetent cells, such as beta lymphocytes, are present in mucous membranes and form a first line of defense. In addition, particles entering with the air are filtered by the nasal mucosa. The cleansing mechanism functions well as long as there is proper gelation in the membranes and the temperature in the nasal cavities remains normal. Temperatures in excess of 107 degrees or much below 64 degrees reduce or shut down the cleansing functions. The same is true for the effectiveness of immune cells. Remaining in overheated or extremely dry rooms for long periods of time in winter is a common prelude to upper respiratory infections.

Insufficient immune response makes the body susceptible to developing a cold. It is actually triggered in over 90 percent of all cases by viruses—mainly rhino and, more seldom, corona viruses. The colloquial use of "strep throat" and "staph infection" have conditioned many into thinking that most simple infections of everyday life are caused by bacteria. This is not correct. However, colds mostly triggered by viruses can be complicated by secondary infections through bacteria that cause inflammations in all organs of the respiratory tract.

In addition, cold, overheated, or moist feet transmit messages through the vegetative nervous system, reducing circulation in the mucous membranes, thereby lowering the oxygen supply and lowering the antibodies in the mucosa. Other factors can also have an impact: a bronchial system damaged from multiple viral, inflammative lung problems; long-lasting or excessive antibiotic therapies that damage the flora in the intestines; alcohol abuse; constant physical or psychological stress; or age-related lack of sexual and adrenal hormones.

Aromatherapy is not directed exclusively at bacteria, which are not even the cause of the problem, but addresses the circumstances that led to a depressed immune system. Essential oils inhibit viral pathogens and improve immune parameters and immunoglobulin levels. Using oils for common colds is a safe and proven method of minimizing symptoms, preventing secondary or super infections, and, in general, supporting the body in fending off the disease. Overcoming infections with the help of herbal remedies and essential oils alone (without the use of antibiotics) leaves the body in a state of improved immune competence. In the holistic view of aromatherapy, miraculous, one-day cures are not the goal, but a support of the body's defense system in achieving a complete healing through reestablished immunocompetence. This can entail going through an infection process for a number of days to strengthen the body. The reward for this endeavor is a strengthened immune system and better health.

Table13.3: Oils for upper respiratory conditions

Oils	**Condition/property**	**Method**
Eucalyptus radiata and *Eucalyptus dives*	Mucolytic and expectorant	Inhalations and chest and back rubs
Eucalyptus globulus		As an alternative to the above
Bay Laurel	Lymphatic support	Three to ten drops applied topically over lymph nodes
Niaouli (MQV)		Preventive, strengthening shower application with ten to twenty drops of the oil
Rosemary, verbenone type	blocked sinuses and stuffy nose	one drop internally, supporting digestive action
Myrtle	bronchial infections	on the skin in rubs, shower (very soft yet effective alternative to the Eucalyptus applications)
Thyme, thujanol type	severe infections	rubs and internal application (quite useful because it combines very broad and forceful antiseptic action with an extremely high tolerability, can be applied repeatedly without irritation of the skin or membranes of the mouth)
Ravensara aromatica	viral infections, flu symptoms, bone pain, fatigue	internally, inhalation, rubs

Preventive measures are most effective when the first glimmers of cold or flu symptoms are noticed. Using *Eucalyptus radiata, Eucalyptus globulus,* and, very importantly, bay laurel in the shower delivers relatively high concentrations of essential oil molecules to the body. This can be combined with a sauna session in which bay laurel is applied topically over the lymph nodes. Up to ten drops of bay laurel may be used in one session. Individuals without particularly sensitive skin may use up to twenty drops per session. This is a treatment that can be repeated, sensibly, during times of increased risk of cold or flu. It should *not* be done on an ongoing basis, as the skin can develop a sensitivity toward bay laurel oil. Application in the shower and sauna can be complemented with inhalation with "nasal straws," described on page 222. Here is an effective mix of oils to use on the nasal straw:

3 parts peppermint
1 part thyme, thymol type
1 part tea tree
1 part lavender
1 part sage

Bronchitis

Symptoms: deep, chesty cough.
Aromatherapy approach: Eucalyptus radiata, Eucalyptus globulus, MQV, *Inula graveolens,* rosemary verbenone.
The aim of the bronchitis treatment is to loosen mucus in the bronchial passages and to stimulate its elimination with mucolytic essential oils. This should be followed up with expectorant oils (*Eucalyptus radiata* and *Eucalyptus globulus* are also effective against the viruses causing bronchitis). Oils can be applied to the chest, over the whole body, or be inhaled. Alternating oils is more effective and pleasant than the repeated use of one oil or the same combination.
Effectiveness: aromatherapy treatments for a fully developed bronchitis offers no miracle cures, but it stimulates sustained im-

provement by preventing bacterial secondary infections. (Most cases of bronchitis are caused by viruses.)

Common cold

Symptoms: runny nose, watery eyes.

Avoid counterproductive measures such as aspirin, ibuprofen, and acetaminophen, and especially needless antibiotic prescriptions.

Aromatherapy approach: Eucalyptus radiata, ravensara aromatica.

Use MQV to strengthen immune responses, and green myrtle as an expectorant and a mood-lightening agent during the depressive days of the cold.

Effectiveness: no wonder cures, as the body must get rid of the virus. Aromatherapy, however, manages the condition and prevents the occurrence of complicating secondary bacterial infections.

Supporting measures: vitamin C.

Rhinitis

Symptoms: stuffy, runny nose, nasal discharge or obstruction.

Aromatherapy approach: nose drops of .25 percent *Inula graveolens,* 2 percent *Calophyllum inophyllum,* .25 percent rosemary verbenone.

Effectiveness: mucolytic oils can be very effective in decongesting nasal passages. Care has to be taken to use oils in concentrations low enough to avoid additional irritation. Interestingly, mucolytic essential oils often cure most effectively when applied in concentrations at or below the threshold of odor detectability.

Supporting measures: vitamin C, beta carotene, homeopathic *Allium cepa.*

Sinusitis

Symptoms: sinus pain, congestion, nasal discharge, fever.

Aromatherapy approach: inhalation of *Eucalyptus radiata* and *Euca-*

lyptus globulus; topical application of rosemary verbenone and *Inula graveolens* in *Calophyllum* and hazelnut oil.

Effectiveness: application of small amounts of rosemary verbenone directly in the nostrils may also be very effective. Caution: This application may be too forceful for some individuals. Careful experimentation is necessary to determine whether this action will be appropriately tolerated by your body.

Supporting measures: Echinacea purpurea, beta carotene, vitamin C.

Tonsillitis/Sore throat

Symptoms: painfully enlarged glands, sore throat.

Aromatherapy approach: at the first signs, take a drop of cypress frequently (in the beginning, every fifteen minutes, later in increasing intervals). For acute tonsillitis, the strong antibacterial oils of savory, oregano, or thyme thymol are appropriate. The best way to safely apply these irritant oils is to put one drop on a charcoal tablet, which is then allowed to slowly disintegrate in the mouth. This way only a minute amount of oil is liberated continuously, and irritation of the membranes by these oils is prevented. For children, these oils should not be given orally, however, they can be massaged into the soles of the feet.

Supporting measures: homeopathic belladonna, *Apis mellifica,* Mercurius.

Common conditions

Acne

Symptoms: pimples, often infected, occurring on the face, back, and/or shoulders. Scars resulting from constant skin eruptions.

Aromatherapy approach: peppermint oil capsules to stimulate elimination of toxins by the liver. Application of thyme linalool, lavender, MQV, and tea tree oils on the affected areas. Using these relatively mild essential oils on the skin can go a long way toward restoring hygiene and stimulating the formation of new and healthy tissue. Rosemary verbenone and rose hip seed oil can be integrated into topical formulas.

Effectiveness: good successes with aromatherapy are achieved if dietary changes are integrated. Acne is an emergency elimination of toxins through the skin. This happens when the liver and kidneys suffer from toxic overload and no longer eliminate sufficiently.

Supporting measures: zinc and vitamin A twice daily before meals; vitamin E 400 IU twice daily before meals. Avoidance of dairy products and pesticide- or hormone-treated foods.

Conjunctivitis

Applications for the eyes present special needs. Essential oils are never to be applied in the eyes. An elegant alternative is presented by the use of aromatic hydrosols. Aromatic hydrosols are the byproduct of the steam distillation process and contain the water soluble, volatile components of the plant that often gives them a fragrance quite like the essential oil but not as strong. Their composition is different from that of the essential oil: richer in water-compatible components and free of very lipophilic substances such as terpene hydrocarbons. This means highly tolerable, antiinflammative, and antiseptic substances are found in aromatic hydrosols, eminently useful for aromatherapy treatments, especially for children when the use of the essential oil might be too strong.

Symptoms: red, swollen, watering eyes, pinkeye.

Aromatherapy approach: add three to five drops fresh lemon juice to a three-ounce bottle of myrtle water (aromatic hydrosol of *Myrtus communis*), spray directly into eye every hour.

Effectiveness: myrtle water is a precious addition to the wealth of aromatherapy remedies, as it is antiseptic and antiallergic and will be effective in most cases of occasional conjunctivitis. For children, awareness of hygiene is also important. In cases of chronic and recurrent conjunctivitis, the effectiveness of myrtle water has been observed to decline, as the deeper causes were not identified or were difficult to avoid (stresses or environmental problems in the workplace).

Earaches

Symptoms: ear pain.

Aromatherapy approach: using aromatherapy is one way to avoid antibiotics for this common childhood condition. Place one to two drops of *Eucalyptus radiata* on a cotton swab and insert it very gently into the ear canal. Thyme linalool type and spike lavender in carrier may be used topically around the ear.

Effectiveness: for this recurring childhood problem, aromatherapy is best integrated with other measures, to best find the road to recovery. Reasonable help during acute states may be expected.

Supporting measures: ear drops from tincture of *Plantago major*, vita min C, zinc, homeopathic pulsatilla, and belladonna. Avoidance of dairy products.

Fever

Symptoms: body temperature higher than 98.6.

Aromatherapy approach: oral application of German chamomile and frankincense.

Effectiveness: the effects of higher molecular components of frankincense are well researched. The internal application of German chamomile during the acute stages of flu is useful because it detoxifies metabolic wastes from pathogenic microorganisms. Note: riding out the storm and not giving in to the temptation of conventional medicine will lead to true healing.

Supporting measures: foot wraps with cold, wet towels.

Fungal contamination of room air

Symptoms: moldy smell.

Aromatherapy approach: for decontamination blend equal parts savory, geranium, palmarosa, and tea tree in a diffuser.

Effectiveness: effectiveness against room-air microorganisms was one of the first properties of essential oils that was very thoroughly documented by science in the mid-1950s. Essential oils diffused into houses and room air contaminated fungal spores, effectively destroying microorganisms and reducing the resulting allergies.

Supporting measures: fresh air and dry conditions if possible.

Lymphatic support

Symptoms: Stagnation of the lymphatic system is associated with a variety of symptoms, stemming from insufficient elimination of toxins.

Aromatherapy approach: topical application of bay laurel over all areas of lymph nodes. The immediate sensation of relief suggests that this procedure is also supportive in flu treatments. Ingestion of one drop of bay laurel, sufficient to cover the linings of the mouth and throat, is also a good way to stop the onset of a sore throat.

Effectiveness: the broad usefulness of bay laurel oil is in stark contrast to the lack of literature on its benefits. Effectiveness is concluded from the sensation of relief and from the abundance of anecdotal evidence.

Supporting measures: none needed.

Reactions to antibiotics

Symptoms: intestinal problems, allergies, irritation, depression, rash, yeast infection, chronic cough, chronic earache.

Aromatherapy approach: ingestion of *Origanum compactum* or *Thymus vulgaris thujanol* is the most direct way to stimulate the recovery of the body's own defense system. Casual ongoing use of mild but invigorating essential oils such as thyme linalool, MQV, *Eucalyptus radiata,* tea tree, and palmarosa is a reasonable way to stimulate a healthy equilibrium in the metabolism. Application of larger amounts of these oils (twenty drops) distributed over the skin after a shower is a preferred and nonintrusive method of application.

Effectiveness: Aromatherapy is probably the modality best suited to render the use of antibiotics unnecessary.

Supporting measures: Lactobacillus acidophilus, Lactobacillus bifidus, vitamins A, E, C, and B.

Digestive tract

Intestinal complaints

The strongly antimicrobial substances of aromatherapy such as cinnamic aldehyde, eugenol, and carvacrol are quite effective in cleansing the intestinal tract of pathogenic bacteria. Recent research has shown that these substances have an even broader effect than has been assumed. They act against the pathogenic bacteria and they mitigate the inflammative processes in the intestines.[1]

These aromatic substances act favorably and distinctly different than antibiotics that destroy the flora in the intestinal tract. After a course of antibiotics, the intestinal flora is open to the onslaught of new microorganisms and to the development of highly unbalanced or unhealthy compositions of bacterial flora. So-called good bacteria such as acidophilus and bifidus are able to metabolize the phenylpropanoids of essential oils. Pathogenic bacteria such as klebsiella or E. coli are destroyed by them. This is a perfect example for the superior and noiseless technologies that evolution has produced.

Complaints of the digestive tract are often an expression of autonomic nervous system imbalances (see below) manifesting in enzyme deficiencies. Rosemary stimulates the metabolic functions of the liver. To be genuine, rosemary has to come from nonindustrial sources. This is best assured by using rosemary verbenone. Tarragon oil perhaps has the most pronounced beneficial action on a stress-plagued digestive tract. An effective synergy to stimulate digestion is cypress, rosemary verbenone, small amounts of peppermint, and anise seed. To stimulate digestion with a spasmolytic component, a combination of rosemary verbenone, basil, peppermint, and anise seed is effective. To emphasize detoxification, use rosemary verbenone, *Thyme thymol,* coriander seed, and bay laurel. To stimulate the digestive tract and cardiovascular activity (after overeating), an effective remedy is a blend of rosemary verbenone, *Helichrysum,* cypress, and tarragon. To support digestion after a bout of too much fat in the diet, blend sage, cypress, and rosemary verbenone.

Diarrhea

Symptoms: diarrhea, sometimes accompanied by nausea. May be caused by bacteria, viruses, fungi, or parasites.

Aromatherapy approach: for the self-medicating individual, determination of the pathogen is often not possible. Cinnamon bark oil can be used alone or in conjunction with oregano oil to take aim at an extremely broad range of pathogenic bacteria. It is well tolerated internally. For bacterial intestinal infections, which can often be identified by their quick and violent onset, oils that often are treacherous to use on the skin such as cinnamon bark and clove are very useful. Their internal application is usually safe and effective, provided they are used in the appropriately small dosage of one drop per application. The best way to ingest these oils is to dilute one drop of the oil into one tablespoon of edible oil (hazelnut or olive) and ingest that mixture in a gelatin capsule. Cypress oil may also be used to slow down a case of diarrhea, yet its effect is marginal compared to that of either *Lactobacillus acidophilus* or *Lactobacillus bifidus* preparations.

Effectiveness: these acute infections seem rare in Western industrial countries. Treatment with essential oils generally works quite well.

Supporting measures: Lactobacillus acidophilus and *Lactobacillus bifidus.*

Table 13.4: Oils for internal conditions

Oil	**Action**
Bay Laurel (*Laurus nobilis)*	anti-putrid
Cinnamon leaf (*Cinnamomum verum)*	anti-infectious
German Chamomile (*Matricaria recutita)*	antiulcerative
Everlast (*Helichrysum angustifolium)*	anti-inflammative
Lemon (*Citrus limon)*	hepatic decongestant
Mastic (*Pistacia lentiscus)*	anti-hemorrhage, integrity of tissue
Peppermint (*Mentha piperita)*	liver regeneration, secretory stimulant
Petitgrain (*Citrus aurantium)*	anti-inflammative
Rosemary verbenone (*Rosmarinus officinalis verbenone)*	liver protection, restores, balances flora
Rockrose (*Cistus ladaniferus)*	anti-hemorrhagic, astringent
Sage (thujone) (*Salvia officinalis)*	corrects flora, antiputrid, regenerating
Savory (*Satureja montana)*	anti-infectious, corrects flora
Tea Tree (*Melaleuca alternifolia)*	anti-infectious, gram (-)
Thyme thymol (*Thymus vulgaris* thymol)	anti-infectious, corrects flora

Degenerative processes in the intestinal tract and Crohn's Disease

Symptoms: frequent, foul-smelling, and soft stools due to an infectious syndrome of the intestinal mucosa and a resulting imbalance in intestinal flora.

Aromatherapy approach: Oral and/or percutaneous application of essential oils influences the improvement of certain symptoms and leads to equilibrium in the colon.

Effectiveness: These conditions are usually slow to respond to treatment with essential oils. It can help to maintain the status quo, ideally until changes in lifestyle or orientation improve the basic disposition of the individual.

Supporting measures: Lactobacillus acidophilus and Lactobacillus bifidus. TCM.

Urogenital tract and STDs

Genital Warts

Symptoms: A variety of wart appearing mostly in the moist parts of the genital or anal areas.

Aromatherapy approach: Papilloma virus infection and associated genital warts can be treated with the essential oil of *Eucalyptus polybractea* chemotype cryptone. In this case, the monoterpene ketone is credited for a large part of the activity against the virus. *Eucalyptus polybractea* chemotype cryptone is used in a 10 percent concentration in a base of *Calophyllum inophyllum*. Hulled viruses are sensitive to essential oils with a monoterpene alcohol/phenol/cineole synergy and naked (nonenveloped) viruses are sensitive to essential oils with a large proportion of terpenoid-ketones.

Effectiveness: Practitioners in the U.S. have reported only sketchy successes with this treatment.

Bladder infection/Cystitis

Symptoms: burning pain on urination.

Aromatherapy approach: recurrent urinary tract infections are often associated with antibiotic-resistant bacteria. The aromatherapy treatment is simple and effective: two drops of tea tree oil, internally, every twenty minutes for the first four to six hours of the treatment. In very resistant cases, one drop of *Origanum compactum* every hour, maximum four times. Caution: Only to be used in ways known to be tolerated by the individual. Baths with MQV and tea tree or rose oil are another option. Use of MQV with daily showers helps to strengthen the whole organism. Tea tree is excellent to treat the first and painful stages of a bladder infection.

Effectiveness: In the case of simple cystitis, excellent.

Supporting measures: cranberry juice, ingestion of acidophilus in liquid or capsule form after meals, elimination of alcohol and tobacco.

Chlamydia

Symptoms: Chlamydia are the most commonly sexually transmitted microorganisms. They cause a non-characteristic primary effect and often go undetected for long periods of time before they cause more serious conditions like edema of the lymphatic system.

Aromatherapy approach: Thymus vulgaris, thuyanol-4 chemotype, used externally and internally over a course of three weeks.

Effectiveness: Given the lack of conventional treatments this moderately effective treatment is still a good choice.

Supporting measures: Vaginal douches with aromatic hydrosols.

The skin and Helichrysum italicum

The story of the essential oil of *Helichrysum italicum* is a perfect example of how a few individuals acting decisively can make a difference in the world. Essential-oil catalogs prior to the early 1980s do not list *Helichrysum italicum.* Today, *Helichrysum* oil (also known as "everlast" or "immortelle") is offered on virtually every ambitious aromatherapy list. The essential oil of *Helichrysum italicum* ssp *serotinum* got its initial boost, at least in American aromatherapy, from Pierre Franchomme and Daniel Pénoël—its use was popularized by their contribution to the Aromatherapy Course of Pacific Institute of

Aromatherapy. Its effects are so convincing that it has never met with any kind of criticism despite the absence of data on its effectiveness. *Helichrysum* oil demonstrates that anecdotal evidence can create a reality without the help of industrially sponsored science.

Helichrysum is more predictable in its action than almost any other oil and is produced and sold by small enterprises that understand the needs of the aromatherapy market. Corporate manipulations are absent. Because of the small amounts offered and the willingness of the importers to pay a fair price to the producers, *Helichrysum italicum* oil is available in its authentic form.

Helichrysum is the appropriate oil for larger injuries until professional care is available. Ideally undiluted, *Helichrysum* oil is administered onto the injury before it is bandaged for a trip to the doctor's office. It will disinfect the wound and, unlike other disinfecting agents, will not be painful. *Helichrysum* oil prevents swelling and inflammation. The formation of new tissue to close the wound is greatly accelerated. Unfortunately, an injury is often necessary to realize the benefits of this oil. Note: *Helichrysum italicum* must be 100 percent genuine and authentic for it to work.

Generally, *Helichrysum italicum* works for all conditions in which inflamed tissue needs to be calmed down and regenerated. *Helichrysum*'s legendary usefulness for the treatment of scars, old or new, resulting from injury or surgery is best trapped by the following synergy: 1 percent *Helichrysum*, 15 percent flax seed oil, and 84 percent of a base oil, preferably hazelnut oil. In the case of cosmetic surgery, the mixture can be applied to the scar starting about a week after the operation. Recoveries have been phenomenal. Apply two to three times per day for about three to six months to see significant results.

Because everlast *(Helichrysum italicum)* oil is so mild, it can be applied undiluted when immediate relief is needed to minimize pain after injuries. A good way to potentiate the effect of the oil in the treatment of bruises and other sports injuries is to apply it in combination with Comfrey cream, which in this case is used as a carrier.

Allergic skin reactions

Symptoms: Suddenly appearing rashes of varying intensity.

Aromatherapy approach: Moroccan chamomile *(Tanacetum annuum)* and everlast, 2 percent in base oil.

Effectiveness: Excellent.

Supporting measures: None needed.

Burns

Symptoms: Redness, partial disintegration of the outer layers of the skin.

Aromatherapy approach: immediate application of true lavender and ice. Even more effective is the application of the proper (-) alpha bisabolol chemotype of German chamomile with ice.

Effectiveness: for minor local burns this is a highly effective way to preserve skin and reduce pain.

Supporting measures: None needed.

Hematoma

Symptoms: black-and-blue discoloration of the skin and possibly swelling.

Aromatherapy approach: a singularly successful treatment is available with *Helichrysum italicum.* Results are sensational. If applied immediately after the incident, the formation of a hematoma can usually be prevented. If applied later, the healing is sped up significantly.

Effectiveness: excellent.

Supporting measures: None needed.

Hemorrhoids

Symptoms: Painfully swollen or ruptured rectal veins.

Aromatherapy approach: a blend of everlast and German chamomile in sesame oil can calm acute hemorrhoidal pain. The essential oils should not exceed 3 percent of the total mixture. A treatment to contract the blood vessels in a chronic but not acutely painful state is cypress, *Helichrysum*, niaouli, and mastic oil in sesame oil.

Effectiveness: variable.

Supporting measures: Strengthening of the circulatory tract according to individual constitution.

Scars/Cheloids

Symptoms: excess tissue.

Aromatherapy approach: Helichrysum, Calophyllum, and rosemary verbenone in rose hip seed and hazelnut oil. Can be used on scars of any size and any age.

Effectiveness: Surprisingly effective if used regularly over time.

Supporting measures: None needed.

Stretch marks

Symptoms: stringy marks and discoloration after pregnancy or weightloss.

Aromatherapy approach: existing stretch marks are treated with *Helichrysum* and flax seed oil in hazelnut oil. To prevent stretch marks, a blend of neroli and cypress in hazelnut can be massaged into the skin during pregnancy.

Effectiveness: generally good.

Supporting measures: Physical activity such as yoga, etc.

Tendinitis

Symptoms: inflammation following overextention of the tendons.

Aromatherapy approach: a combination of *Helichrysum*, yarrow, and *Eucalyptus citriodora,* ideally applied in base of Comfrey cream, can offer relief if used regularly.

Effectiveness: Moderate but useful in an otherwise difficult situation.

Supporting measures: Comfrey creme.

Wounds and cuts

Symptoms: Small wounds, papercuts and larger up to gashing injuries.
Aromatherapy approach: wounds and cuts can receive an emergency treatment with either some drops of lavender oil, put directly onto the wound, or, if the injuries are bigger, undiluted *Helichrysum* and/or tea tree.
Effectiveness: Immediate pain relief.
Supporting measures: None needed if professional help can be obtained quickly.

Viral infections

Essential oils counteract viral diseases gently and effectively by inhibiting the pathogen and by improving the overall metabolic ac-

Table 13.5: Historic developments that led to an understanding of viruses

1800s	Charles Chaimberland invented a porcelain filter that bacteria were unable to penetrate. Dimitrii Ivanovski observed that agents causing tobacco mosaic disease were able to penetrate such a filter.
1911	Peyton Ross showed that a filtrate that was free of cells could induce malignant growths in animals. Only entities other than bacteria were assumed to be in the filtrate.
1915	The smallest known organisms, bacteria, were shown to be subject to invasion by even smaller entities.
Mid-1920s	cell-culture techniques were implemented to study the effects of viruses upon the living cell.
1940	The first direct observation of viruses became possible through the electron microscope. Previously, viruses were only defined by their small size.
1952	The He-La cell line was initiated and has since served as a very useful cell culture to study the behavior of viruses.

tivity and immune response. Essential oils improve the emotional well-being and advance the healing of the immuno-psychological aspects of viral diseases.

Viruses are infectious subcellular particles. They consist of DNA or RNA: genetic material surrounded (in the case of "hulled" viruses) by a protein or lipoprotein "coat." This hull protects the nucleic acid and also provides, in different ways, for the virus' ability to invade other cells. Viruses are independent genetic systems that take over the cell's machinery, causing it to synthesize virus-protein and virus-nucleic acid. Viruses are not organisms. They can only replicate themselves in the living cell, which, being infected, produces new virus-nucleic acid and according to that blueprint synthesizes the envelope proteins. Their replication within the living cell and transfer through infection cause characteristic reactions in the host cell and in the host organism.

Experience and research suggest that essential oils that contain either strongly electrophilic (phenols or terpene alcohols) or strongly nucleophilic (citral) constituents are most effective in

Table 13.6: Essential oils effective for treatment of viral conditions

Essential oils	**Synergy**
Ravensara aromatica, Laurus nobilis, Eucalyptus radiata, niaouli	alpha-terpineol/cineole
tea tree *(Melaleuca alternifolia)* and *Melaleuca linariifolia*	terpineol-4/cineole
Eucalyptus globulus	pinocarveol/cineole
spike lavender	linalool/cineole

treating diseases caused by hulled viruses. Particular effectiveness has been found with essential oils with a built-in synergy of terpene alcohols and cineole (such as *Ravensara aromatica*).

The suggested mode of treatment of viral conditions is a combination of mainly external applications of the essential oils. A one-to-one combination of ravensara and *Eucalyptus radiata* is an effective blend for liberal topical application. The oil combination is used for four aerosol sessions per five to ten minutes of inhalation per day. For transcutaneous use, the oil blend should be rubbed on the thorax several times per day, if necessary every half hour, using up to 1/2 oz. during a day. One drop of *Lavandula spica* chemotype linalool can be taken internally every half hour (in a teaspoon of honey).

Epstein-Barr virus

Considerable success in treating Epstein-Barr virus symptoms are generally reported by practitioners with basically the same strategy as outlined above. The treatments include supporting liver functions (peppermint and *Thymus vulgaris* thuyanol type internally). The oils reportedly remedy much of the usual fatigue associated with these conditions.

Flu

Symptoms: fever, muscle aches, headaches, loss of appetite. The onset is often quite sudden. Nasal or bronchial symptoms may occur but are much less common than with the common cold. Influenza is a viral condition, and no effective conventional medical treatment exists to date.

Aromatherapy approach: similar to that of common cold. The dosages applied may be high, and are mainly delivered topically and through inhalation. For broad effects, *Thyme thuyanol* and geraniol types may be used. Spike lavender and green myrtle can be integrated to prevent complications such as pneumonia. *Ravensara aromatica,* applied topically or ingested (two drops every two hours), energizes during the most acute and debilitating days of a flu. German chamomile may be taken internally to help the body detoxify the metabolic wastes of proliferating microorganisms as well as reduce fever.

Effectiveness: prevention of secondary infection, maintenance of emotional stability, and functionability can usually achieved. No wonder cures are available, though. However, going through a flu cycle with the help of essential oils and other natural measures will usually strengthen the body through the avoidance of ineffective antibiotics and the associated immune depression.

Supporting measures: vitamin C, multivitamins, and healthy nutrition.

Pénoël claims that an aromatic treatment of a viral condition begun right at the onset cuts the disease on the first day.

The fast action of the aromatic treatment is a result of the direct inhibition of the virus through the essential oil and the powerful effect on the host, or terrain, in which the pathogen exists. Essential oils alter the pH as well as (electrical) resistance of humoral fluids in a way that is adverse to the virus, and they induce higher levels of immunoglobulin A.

Intensive treatments should produce significant improvements within two or three days. If this is not the case, a new selection of essential oils may be required, or a reassessment of the illness. Reassessment is also necessary if bacterial superinfections occur, in which case antibacterial essential oils should also be used. If inflammative processes are prevailing, essences with a high proportion of aldehydes will be effective (combining antiviral with antiinflammative effects). If dry mucus needs to be liquefied, essences with a high proportion of ketones will be required. All in all, the use of essential oils should allow a highly appropriate management of a flu virus. The results are usually quick and lasting.

Proper nutrition is an important factor in the treatment of almost every condition. The healing and health-maintaining influence of the right foods, and the detrimental effects of junk food and pesticide- or hormone-loaded food cannot be overestimated. Helpful literature such as *Healing with Whole Foods*, by Paul Pitchford, should be consulted by every health-conscious person.

Herpes simplex

Symptoms: periodic painful lesions around the mouth.

Aromatherapy approach: apply essential oils topically on the lesions, ideally prior to the outbreak in order to prevent the occurrence of full-fledged lesions. Lavender, *Eucalyptus globulus, Eucalyptus citriodora,* geranium, or melissa are highly effective. The recommended course of action is to apply the oils hourly for the first twenty-four hours, if well tolerated undiluted. Once the lesions start to dry out and the skin becomes dry and taut, the application of the oils should be continued in a hazelnut oil base with the addition of vitamin E.

Effectiveness: herpes can be treated with aromatherapy, but you should be under the care of a doctor. Aromatherapy is effective. Recurrence can be frequent using aromatherapy, and often outbreaks can completely be prevented through early application.

Shingles/Herpes zoster

Symptoms: strong nerve pain accompanied by itching red rash in the waist area.

Aromatherapy approach: shingles is a disease treated easily and effectively with aromatherapy by topical application of a fifty-fifty mix of *Calophyllum inophyllum* and *Ravensara aromatica.* The former stimulates phagocytosis. Topical application of this blend of oils effects healing within two days to a week and there is usually no recurrence. Oral use of peppermint three to four times a day is recommended by Pénoël and Franchomme. If the vesicles have disappeared but the pain still persists, frequent application of aromatic hydrosol of Roman chamomile brings relief.

Effectiveness: the treatment of herpes simplex labialis and shingles is generally an excellent success for aromatherapy, especially if the oils are applied as soon as the first symptoms appear. See a doctor immediately, since these are infectious conditions.

Autonomic Nervous System

Stress and the digestive tract

Gastrointestinal-tract problems, stemming from agitation or stress are best addressed with essential oils from culinary herbs such as rosemary, tarragon, or basil. As these herbs are part of our Western culture, we are often able to develop an intuition as to which oil

Table 13.7: Oils for nervousness, tension and stress

Condition	Aromatherapy treatment
Anxiety:	Blend of neroli, mandarin, orange, petitgrain, spikenard; one drop of mixture applied to temples
Tachycardia and hangover:	Anise; one drop in half a glass of water or on a sugar cube
Upset stomach:	Tarragon, rosemary verbenone, marjoram, one or two drops in water
Sedative body oil: (for the evening)	Eucalyptus citriodora or spikenard with lavender. Ten drops in bath tub (or in hazelnut oil for smoother skin)
Restlessness:	Mandarin, everlast, one drop on solarplexus or internally
Trouble falling asleep:	Angelica, three drops on the forehead
Shortness of breath:	Inula graveolens, 10 percent in base oil rubbed on chest and back
Shortness of breath: (caused by tension)	Ammi visnaga, 10 percent in base oil on chest and back
Circulatory stimulation:	Petitgrain and everlast, a drop on sugar cube or rosemary camphor, a drop on sugar cube or vetiver in Hazelnut as a body oil

might work best for a specific problem. Tarragon oil is very effective in restoring balance in stress-related disorders and complaints of spasms. Rosemary can help stimulate slow digestion caused by a lack of digestive enzymes. Anise seed oil will alleviate the unpleasant symptoms of a hangover and stabilize the heart rhythm. Peppermint stimulates stagnant liver activity. Other oils with generally very favorable effect on the digestive tract include coriander, cardamom, and marjoram. Spectacular results can be achieved with the smallest amounts of essential oils.

Cramps and tension

Minimal trial-and-error efforts often result in general relief for a great many different complaints. For general relaxation in baths or during massages, pleasant essences with high ester content provide relief through direct interaction with the central nervous system. Useful choices are clary sage, geranium, and lavender. The general rule for the whole group of stress-related symptoms is to experiment with essential oils to find out which plant works best.

For muscular tension or cramps, Roman chamomile and *Mandarin petitgrain* provide immediate relief. For anxiety, neroli could be an excellent first choice. Depressive states are more difficult, but not impossible, to address with essential oils. The fast action and quick elimination of essential oils are often not sustained enough to provide lasting relief for depressions. But with the availability of more and varied extracts of St. Johnswort, effective treatment can be achieved. Depending on the constitution of the individual, the uniquely uplifting qualities of the nonintrusive *Lemon verbena* can provide immediate amelioration.

Just prior to sleep, different oils such as angelica (three to nine drops massaged on the solar plexus) or cumin (nine drops internally within an hour before bedtime) can be tried. For a more sustained improvement in cases of insomnia, the casual and continuous use of orange, mandarin, and neroli either applied sparingly to the temples or as a perfume in the bedroom should be tried.

Asthma

The number of asthma patients is on the rise, mainly as a result of increasing environmental and emotional stresses. The medical establishment is quite helpless in addressing the real causes. While new and "improved" medications are continuously introduced to the consumer market, the mortality rate of asthma sufferers is still increasing. One look at the serious side-effects that many of these drugs have is enough to observe the strictly symptomatic approach at work here.

A vicious cycle is created for the asthma patient. Physical dependency is created through cortisone and cortisone-like drugs. Psychological dependency is created by the impression or belief that the patient is unable to survive without medication. This can create situations where the individual suffers an attack only by discovering that the "lifesaving" aerosol spray is not within reach.

Symptoms: shortness of breath, inability to breathe.

Aromotherapy approach: Two main categories of patients need to be distinguished: the patient who has had asthma problems over a long period of time and has had allopathic treatments, and the patient who has just started to develop breathing problems and is not yet dependent on allopathic drugs. In the first case, the disease has often developed into a physical problem. Attempts to cure it must proceed in several phases. In the second case, only the first two steps of the aromatherapy approach will often suffice, as the asthma has not yet left its physical imprint on the organs. In this case the symptoms are aroused by stimuli or the emotional/psychological landscape, and supportive, strengthening aromatherapy treatments are adequate and remarkably effective.

Asthma patients need to become acquainted with essential oils slowly and cautiously, especially when they are unfamiliar with natural fragrances. Sometimes a little education helps to familiarize the patient with the olfactory quality of essential oils. Interestingly, people with civilization disorders are often completely used to synthetic fragrance and find the purity of essential oil fragrance overpowering and not at all attractive.

Best suited for such introductory endeavors are gentle, relaxing massages with pleasantly fragrant compositions of antispasmodic essential oils. Light, soothing combinations such as lavender and mandarin are helpful (the often-substituted tangerine does not contain the important antispasmodic agent N-methyl-methylanthranilate), as well as a small amounts of Roman chamomile or strongly antispasmodic blends like spikenard *(Nardostachys jatamansi),* Roman chamomile, mandarin petitgrain, and clary sage.

Asthma patients respond quite well to these essences and begin to build a positive attitude around the use of aromatherapy.

The next recommended step is the liberal use of *Eucalyptus radiata* or *Ravensara aromatica* during a morning shower. These oils, well known for their strong expectorant qualities, show a surprising antiasthmatic effect, which research has shown to be due to their terpene alcohol contents. Provided the asthma patient responds well to these measures, more intensive treatments may be initiated.

For the nervous and allergic type of asthmatic, an antispasmodic and stabilizing blend of tarragon, mandarin *(Citrus reticula),* and rosemary verbenone represents the next level of treatment. This blend may be taken in capsules or used in a diffuser for inhalation. Additionally effective is complementing this treatment with one or more of the oils of cypress, ylang ylang, or Roman chamomile.

Patients in whom the condition has transformed into a combination of chronic bronchitis and asthma, accompanied with a strong physical impairment, can benefit from general stimulation by the ingestion of oregano (capsules of 50 mg or 1–2 drops) *Origanum compactum* in a base of sunflower seed oil).

These treatments can be augmented after about two weeks with a suppository treatment that is specifically suited to combat acute crises. Of course, this must only be done after the patient has positively accepted the oils and has conscientiously decided to utilize the healing potential of aromatherapy. Prepare suppositories in a cocoa butter/coconut oil base with 175 mg (approx. 6 drops) of a blend of *Ammi visnaga* (50 mg (approx. 2 drops)) and *Hyssop* off. var. *decumbens* (125 mg (approx. 4 drops)). Do not use *Hyssop* off. var. *officinalis*, the high ketone content makes it patently unsafe for these applications. The *H. decumbens* variety is practically free of ketones but has a desirably high proportion of the antiasthmatic and tonifying compound trans-linalool-oxide.

Auto-immune problems

Conditions attributed to Epstein-Barr virus, like chronic fatigue syndrome and fibromyalgia have been treated with aromatherapy. Strong immunostimulant essential oils such as oregano, thyme, clove, or, best of all, cinnamon should be used in a tolerable fashion, which means taking frequent small dosages. Cinnamon oil can be dissolved in an edible vegetable oil and ingested in capsule form. The dosage per capsule or per application should not be above 1 to 2 drops. The maximum recommended dosage for these capsules for day one and two of the treatment is 10 x 1 drops (10 drops per day). Using these capsules maybe five or six times a day is sufficient. On the third day, the dosage should be cut in half so that a maximum of 5 x 1 drop per day of oil is taken and the other part being substituted with a single essential oil within the group of the terpene alcohol essential oils: palmarosa, tea tree, or *Ravensara aromatica* are good choices. The variation between essential oils and different mixes of essential oils, all of which should be high in terpene alcohols, will be more effective than the use of a single essential oil to which the body might adjust in a certain way. This rather broadly designed treatment has been implemented in many alternative practice situations and, given the diffuse nature of these conditions, the results were encouraging.

If balancing of the intestinal flora is the goal of the treatment, these stronger essential oils might need to be taken over two to three weeks. These oils are tolerated quite well internally and different practices report different dosages ranging from 1–10 drops of essential oil per day.

Allergies

There are at least two ways of dealing with allergies. In the old paradigm, drugs are used to suppress the symptoms of allergy. The hallmarks of typical allopathic treatments are present when we see patients who are sicker than before they began treatment. Steroids with all their highly detrimental side-effects are used to suppress an overreacting immune system. To achieve real improvement, it is useful to see allergies for what they are: reactions to environmental stimuli, and learned behavior. Through a sequence of events our immune system becomes conditioned to trigger its response with full force when certain agents are present (often pollen of various plants). We sneeze and our eyes water. Often allergies are misread. When reactions to tomatoes occur, our system often is responding to the pesticides the tomatoes have been sprayed with.

The aromatherapy approach can be cumbersome and slow. In fact, some individuals may have such a strong tendency to develop allergic reactions that the oil approach may be too weak to work at all. But there are moderate possibilities at hand. Certain oils contain principles that reduce allergic symptoms. MQV oil and myrtle water are antiallergic. Moroccan chamomile (*Tanacetum annuum*) has antiinflammative and antihistaminic properties. A mixture of MQV, *Tanacetum annuum* and peppermint is a remedy worth trying for symptomatic relief. This mixture may be applied topically and may also be ingested. While this mixture does provide certain relief from allergic symptoms, it is not a miracle cure.

Symptoms: itching, watery eyes, stuffy or congested nose, fever.

Aromatherapy approach: two-thirds-part MQV and one-third-part *Tanacetum annuum* along with three drops peppermint. Mix with cold water and apply to face. Myrtle water may also be applied to the face.

Effectiveness: The self-help aromatherapy approach with essential oils is for the most part cumbersome and unimpressively slow. As a matter of fact some individuals may have such strong tendency to develop allergic reactions that the oil approach may be too weak and simply not working.

Supportive measures: vitamin B; avoid dairy products and food treated with pesticides and hormones.

Arthritis

Symptoms: Generally joint pain.
Aromatherapy approach: 10 drops Eucalyptus citriodora, 10 drops Helichrysum italicum in 5 ml Sesame oil.
Effectiveness: The aromatherapy approach is limited to easing the acute pain with anti-inflammative essences.
Supportive measures: TCM offers herbal mixtures which help detoxification.

Women's Health Issues

Vaginitis

Symptoms: excessive vaginal discharge, bad smell and itching, frequent and painful urination.
Aromatherapy approach: soak a tampon in a blend of: fifty drops tea tree, ten drops *Thymus vulgaris* thymol, and sixty drops hazelnut oil. Leave this in for several hours, three times per day. Also, sit in a bath of warm to hot water with MQV, tea tree, and, if possible, *Inula graveolens.*
Effectiveness: this approach is at least as effective as antibiotic treatment and has no side-effects.
Supportive measures: twice daily, douche with unsweetened unpasteurized yogurt.

PMS and menopause

Premenstrual syndrome (PMS) appears a number of days before the end of the cycle and can cause anxiety, irritability, emotional fluctuations, sleeplessness, headaches, tension, painful swelling of the breasts, bloated abdomen, and edema in the legs and feet. These symptoms result from an increased level of estrogen and depressed levels of progesterone in this part of the cycle.

Symptoms: Premenstrual syndrome (PMS) appears a number of days before the monthly bleeding. Anxiety, irritability, emotional flucuations, sleeplessness, headaches, tension, painful swelling of the breast, bloated abdomen and edema in the legs and feet.

Aromatherapy approach: A new essential oil extracted from a plant that has traditionally been used to alleviate the associated problems of PMS and menopause throughout history has been used in herbal preparations as a tincture. Recently, researchers have tried to isolate one or more active principles that could have progesterone-mimicking character or in some other way could counteract the hormonal deficiencies of PMS. None of these principles were identified in the tinctures. The researchers proceeded to analyze the essential oil of *Vitex agnus castus*. In the oil, no compounds were detected that could be associated with the effects. However, a number of unidentified compounds were found in the oil and in the absence of more conclusive proof, we can assume that those are the ones responsible for the well-known effects of *Vitex*. Indeed, extracts of this plant have a very interesting pharmacology. From previously conducted research and observation of human use it was concluded that the extract of *Vitex* interacts directly with the pituitary gland. One drop per day is taken orally during the second half of the cycle.

Effectiveness: The use of *Vitex* essential oil for PMS is new. The anecdotal evidence gathered in the last two years suggests it is a much more effective treatment than the usual aromatherapy measures.

Supportive measures: If effectiveness is verified on the suggested level, none needed.

"To gather wild azalea,
If you can bear to break,
Is laying by a treasure
For your heart's sake."
—Hildegarde Flanner

Epilogue

Understanding Nature will not give you scientific proof, but it will give you the right answers.

Many of the previously not understood effects of essential oils are explained by the interactions of essential-oil components with receptor systems in the body. Monoterpene hydrocarbons, found in needle oils and elsewhere, stimulate metabolic processes including detoxification and regeneration (mediated by receptor interaction and expression). Oils from many different plants all contain monoterpene hydrocarbon compounds and will all have these effects. Consequently, in many cases aromatherapy is not merely a matter of choosing a specific oil. Individual and specific secondary metabolic products give unique qualities to an essential oil not necessarily found in another oil.

The body's own transmitters, and receptor molecules on the surface and inside cells all over the body, represent an intricate system of communication, sending and receiving a constant stream of emotional and physiological messages. The free flow of this communication is a prerequisite for good health. Essential-oil molecules interact with different sites, triggering different processes. Often different molecules present in one oil trigger seemingly opposing effects. The substances present in one oil generate multiple effects, such as stimulating and acting as a local anesthetic at the same time with the end result being a carefully self-regulating and limiting effect benefiting the whole human being. The resulting overall effects are carefully balanced and truly natural—exemplified for instance in the well-known subtle and multilayered qualities of ginger. This is the reason the interaction with plants will always be superior to that with synthetic substances. The latter are composed of lifeless elements with a one-dimensional principle of action. They may generate a beneficial action in one spot of the human, but what is normally termed undesirable side effects is a representation of the action of that same compound on other aspects of body or metabolism that are detrimental and not tempered or balanced by other synergistic principles. Synthetics are not self-correcting in their action; compared to nature they are primitive.

Future research on these terpene and phenylpropane receptor interactions will provide more such surprising findings, such as the antitumor activity of limonene. At the same time, research results represent bits and pieces of very specific information, which tends to obscure the bigger picture rather than clarify it. It is a daunting task to attempt to uncover every single possible interaction and weigh it against all others occurring at the same time.

More inclusive assessments come from enlightened observation of plants in the tradition of Paracelsus or Goethe. Observing plant organisms, how and where they live, how they function, and what challenges they face will complement the details garnered through test-tube research.

Lipophilic messenger hypothesis revisited

When monoterpenes developed for the first time on a huge global scale as secondary products of needle-tree metabolism, the biochemical engineering of the plants brilliantly integrated two seemingly antagonistic features. Specifically shaped molecules were necessary to interact with receptors, which originally developed in a hydrophilic environment and are geared toward peptides, or at least polar, hydrophilic substances. By making the monoterpenes light and lipophilic, they became volatile and able to travel through air. This way they could not only communicate with the receptors of other organisms, they could also overcome the stationary nature of plants. In short, what makes pinene special is that it interacts with receptors and travels through air.

Today's understanding of the complex, multidimensional processes initiated by odoriferous substances reveals how humans in earlier times must have related to fragrance. Günther Ohloff finds captivating words for the prehistoric fragrance experience:

> Invisible, imponderable, untouchable and, only for a volatile moment, sensually comprehensible, scent must have appeared like a Fata Morgana to prehistoric man. The unfamiliar nothing released feelings and reactions which he had not planned and led to a behavior which he had no control upon. Instinct and scent go through the nose and ensure the survival of the species. So the sense of smell as a relic of the animalistic origin of human beings seems to be the most archaic of all senses. It stands at the beginning of his wisdom—his "nose wisdom." The *Homo sapiens* was originally *Homo odorus*, the "smelling one."[1]

Beginning the journey

The Sumerian culture created concepts in which matter was animated with spirit. In their perfume creations they revealed their purest essence, their spirituality. A small tablet, given with a perfume gift, carried the inscription, "In this little bottle are 100 rose petals from my garden, each one reveals a message of love for you." The Sumerians founded a broad civilization with sciences, literature, astronomy, and architecture. With spiritual interpretations given to flowers and plants, and other objects of their daily affairs, they increased their appreciation of esthetics and imbued their lives with new values. It is not surprising that the Garden of Eden was given to them, as Genesis says: "And Jehovah planted a garden in Eden, in the East between the rivers and the trees with many flowers and fruits, and into it He put the human whom He had created."

Following the Sumerians were the Babylonians, whose rituals often included, according to Herodot, exorbitant amounts of perfumes. The Assyrian culture was one of the most important in Asia Minor from the twelfth to the seventh century B.C. At the time, fifteen different perfumes were known, including narde, cinnamon, saffron, rose, iris root, and aloe. In the gardens, rose, violet, jasmine, iris, saffron, narde, mimosa, hyacinth and narcissus were cultivated. Throughout history, spirituality, medicine, and ritual were connected. Fragrance is inextricably tied to the mysteries of life, to love, to procreation, and to the human search for meaning.

This magical or spiritual ritualistic nature is exemplified in some of the West's most influential historic periods: God told Moses and his people on their exodus from Egypt to take with them hundreds of bags of myrrh, cinnamon, rose, galbanum, and frankincense. Wherever we look in historic writings, myrrh and frankincense and many others have been consistently employed for ritual, healing, transition, and transcendence.

With this in mind it is clear that what is learned today through science about the complexity of sesquiterpenoid substances is only the tip of the iceberg. A new science, not fixed on dead matter, may pull the veil away from the tangible magic that essential oils and fragrances represented throughout history. As discussed, constituents present in myrrh are now known to interact with the psycho-neurological circuits repressing the sensation of pain and binding to the receptors of bliss, the opioid receptors. Similarly, frankincense has been found to be a uniquely effective anti-inflammative agent in specific conditions such as chronic polyarthritis, bronchial asthma, Crohn's disease, and ulcerative colitis. From the flurry of research on sesquiterpenes and receptor interaction, it can be extrapolated that a broad variety of interactions with the psycho-neurological area will be found. Cultural evidence—the linking of fragrances to ritual, magic, transcendence, and consciousness—proved that interactions between plants, animals, and humans are beneficial.

From prehistoric times to War and Peace

The culture of fragrance must have begun long before recorded history, possibly originating from the time humans first made fire. How could the people of this time comprehend the dizzying variety of olfactory impressions that could be had through the burning of different fragrance materials? How could this variety of impressions be interpreted, which were so distinctly different from the fragrance impressions of the environment they were accustomed to? Making fire happened through divine intervention. Smoke ascending to the sky was an offering to the gods for their benevolence. Pleasant fragrances could protect the living and the dead, strengthen the healthy and heal the ill, and connect humans with their ancestors. Tales, myths, and symbols originating long before written scriptures and handed down through oral tradition over the millennia are witness to a blossoming language of fragrance. The first records of this language reach back more than five thousand years.

The Bible has many pointers to the importance of erogenous fragrance. King Solomon, who apparently exerted a strong attraction on women, talks of the fragrances that make his bed and his desires irresistible: myrrh, aloe, and cinnamon. It seems natural that cinnamon oil, stimulating and beneficial to the whole metabolism, also acts as an aphrodisiac via a general enhancement of all body functions.

But it's not only cinnamon that galvanizes the fantasy of philosophers and writers. Plato writes about how the "lost paradise" smelled of ambrosia and other fragrances. In Tolstoy's *War and Peace,* Prince Peter dances with Helena, and is so intoxicated by her fragrance he immediately desires her for himself. Through the message of her perfume it became clear to Peter that Helena had to become his wife, that no other option was possible. Rovesti, a firm believer in the power of smell, finds this somewhat excessive and comments, "Only much later I understood this magic.... And following [my reading of] Tolstoy was an unavoidable period of romantic reading, reaching from Baudelaire, with his many hints on the eroticizing effects of fragrance, to the paradoxical statement of the physiologist, Binet, that for many men, even today, the most important aspect of a woman is not her mind, her beauty, her personality, but her smell." One might add that much of the research discussed in Chapter 2 suggests that the reverse might also be true.

The connection

The complete history of the use of aromatic substances, from ancient ritual and medicinal uses up to the songs of contemporary writers, is testimony that the lipophilic messengers, transmitters, and receptor-based psychosomatic network is as old as humanity. In an era of scientific exploration of the laws of the material world, these connections were overlooked and/or ignored. The material manifestation of these aspects of human life, transmitter molecules, and receptor sites are so enormously effective in such small concentrations that for a long time nobody had a clue that they were there. As a result, everything that could not be proven with the scientific method of the moment was arrogantly dismissed as an old wives tale—an involuntary admission and ironic perpetuation of the warring male model of medicine. In fact the opposite is true: the connections between natural substances and health do exist and do exert the most pronounced influences.

If essential oils are truly made from nature they possess enormous beauty and healing potential. Aromatherapy based on such oils is in sharp contrast to the conventional medical paradigm, which itself is based on the culture of industrialization and alienation. Aromatherapy constitutes a rare and valid alternative to secular medical consumerism.

Visions shows how a future might look when mankind keeps giving in to the fallacy of improving upon nature or playing God.

But the concept of progress is also given new and original thought, expressed in such recent books as *Small is Beautiful, Resurgence of the Real, Spontaneous Healing, Molecules of Emotion,* and *Voice of the Earth*. In these authors' view, a healthy and balanced life is only marginally advanced by science and industrialization.

Balance and good health come from staying within the limits of one's own body, mind, and soul and understanding the spiritual reconstruction needed to overcome the violent consequences of the epidemic of emptiness. Aromatherapy contributes, however modestly, to these ends. It is of assistance whenever the individual psychosomatic network needs support. It is the key for *Homo scientificus* to approach the intensely complex, subtle, powerful, noiseless, and effective chemistry of nature not only with the limiting view of material science but also through the higher planes of human consciousness that incorporates awe and respect for the phenomenon of life.

Glossary

Absolute: Fragrance material obtained by solvent extraction of flowers or plants. This method is used in particular to extract fragrance materials which do not withstand the heat of distillation or for plants with a very low yield of fragrance material.

Acetylcholine: A neurotransmitter active in the autonomic nervous system.

Adrenaline: A messenger substance produced by the adrenal glands.

Aflatoxin: A fungal toxin with a coumarin structure.

Angiosperm: Plant with seeds enclosed in a fruit, grain, pod, or capsule.

Antihistamine: Any of various substances used to block the action of histamine compounds released from human tissues during allergic reactions.

Aromachology: The scientific study of the psychological effects of fragrance.

Biosynthetic pathway: A sequence of biochemical steps which generate natural substances.

Camphor: An aromatic ketone compound found in many essential oils. One of the first compounds whose chemical structure was understood.

Chemical family: Mostly named after the functional group attached to terpenoid molecular skeletons. The attachment of a functional group to a basic hydrocarbon molecule influences its pharmacology greatly. Compounds with identical functional groups fall into the same chemical family and share similar pharmacological properties.

Chemical race: Populations of one species which differ in their chemical make-up from other populations of the same species.

Chemotype: A plant with a chemical composition distinct from others of the same species.

Chloroplast: The parts of a cell able to perform photosynthesis.

Complementary medicine: Modalities perceived as holistic or natural.

Enantiomers/Enantiomeric: Mirror-image isomers, identical chemical compounds composed of the same kinds and numbers of atoms differing only in their symmetry.

Endocrine system: The human glandular system responsible for the secretion of hormones (chemical messengers) into the blood and lymphatic system.

Episiotomy: Incision of the perineum to prevent rupture when giving birth.

Eucaryotes: Organisms with a true nucleus (including chromosomes) in their cells.

Farnesyl pyrophosphate: Physiological form of the precursor to sesquiterpenes.

Fractionated distillation: Separating a mixture through repeated distillation.

Frontal cortex: The most forward of the outer layer of the brain, present only in primates. It contains neuronal centers for language, conceptualization, judgment and contemplation.

Geranyl pyrophosphate: Physiological form of the precursor to terpenes.

Hysterectomy: Surgical excision of the uterus. So named because this was once considered an effective treatment for hysteria.

Isomer: Chemical compounds composed of the same kinds and numbers of atoms but with different structural arrangements.

Isoprene: A five carbon molecule. Precursor to terpenoid molecules.

Kidney epithelium: Exterior kidney tissue.

Ligand: Molecules which bind to specific sites. In molecular biology molecules which attach to receptor sites and convey messages to the cell.

Lipophilic: Literally, lipid or fat-loving, as in essential oil molecules which dissolve in fats and oils.

Mastectomy: Surgical excision of the breast.

Mitochondria: The "power plant" of the cell, performing many metabolic functions.

Nature identical: Implies that molecules of a synthetic odorant are identical to the make-up of natural odorants. In reality the composition of natural odorants is always more complex than the synthetic look-alike.

Osteoporosis: A loss of bone tissue, leaving the overall shape of the bones intact yet rendering them increasingly porous, brittle, and subject to fracture.

Oxygenated terpenoids: 10-carbon essential oil constituents with side chains which contain oxygen and oxygen-containing compounds.

Peptide: Chains of amino acids.

Phenylpropanoid: Molecules derived from a basic 9-carbon structure of a (6 carbon) phenyl ring system with an attached side chain of 3 carbons.

Phytotherapy: The medicinal uses of plants. Aromatherapy is a branch of phytotherapy.

Procaryote: One celled-organisms without the more specialized features of eucaryotes.

Receptor: A molecule anchored in the outer cell membrane with a site accessible to ligands such as hormones, drugs or neurotransmitters.

Shikimic acid: Biological precursor to phenylpropanoids.

Steroid: Natural steroids are derivates of the terpenoid biosynthetic pathway and cholesterol, including sex- and adrenal hormones.

Symbiosis: The mutually beneficial living together of two organisms.

Symmetrical: Perfect equality of proportion and form, as in a mirror image.

Synapse: A region where nerve impulses are transmitted from one nerve cell to another.

Terpene: Basic 10-carbon molecules which characterize most essential oils. Aroma and pharmacology of terpenes are fundamental for aromatherapy.

Triterpene: A molecule with a 30-carbon structure, not usually found in volatile essential oils.

Volatile: Easily evaporates.

WONF: Acronym for "With Other Natural Flavors". Includes substances which originate from natural chemicals but have been chemically altered.

References

Chapter One

1. Hänsel, Rudolf. 1993. Therapeutische Anwendung Ätherischer Öle. In *Ätherische Öle, Anspruch und Wirklichkeit,* Carle, Reinhold (ed), 203-230. Wissenschaftliche Verlagsgesellschaft mbH, Stuttgart.
2. Buchbauer, G. 1992. Biological Effects of Fragrances and Essential Oils. In *Proceedings of the 12th International Congress of Flavors, Fragrances and Essential Oils,* Woidich, H. and Buchbauer, G. (eds), 456-461. Austrian Assoc. Flav. Fragr. Industry, Vienna.
   —Buchbauer, G. Jäger, W., Nasel, B., Ilmberger, J. and Dietrich, H. 1994. The Biology of Essential Oils and Fragrance Compounds. Aromatherapy Symposium, Essential Oils, Health & Medicine, November 18-20. White Plains, New York.
3. Gattefossé, Réné Maurice. 1993. *Gattefossé's Aromatherapy.* C.W. Daniel Company Limited, Saffron Walden, UK.
4. Valnet, Jean. 1980. *The Practice of Aromatherapy.* Destiny Books, New York.
5. Tisserand, Robert. 1977. *The Art of Aromatherapy.* Healing Arts Press, Rochester, VT.
6. Belaiche, Paul. 1979. *Traite de phytotherapie et d'aromatherapie.* Maloine S.A. Editeur, Paris.
7. Franchomme, Pierre and Pénoël, Daniel. 1990. *L'aromathérapie éxactement.* Roger Jollois Editeur, Limoges.

8. Viaud, Henri. 1983. *Huiles Essentielles—Hydrolats, Distillation, Qualité, Contrôle de la Pureté, Indications Majeures.* Editions PRÉSENCE, Sisteron, France.
9. Kusmirek, J. 1992. Defining Aromatherapy. In *Perfumery: The Psychology and Biology of Fragrance,* van Toller, S. and Dodd, G. H. (eds) 277. Elsevier Science Publishers Ltd. Essex.
10. Kaku, Michio. 1997. *Visions.* 192. Doubleday, New York.
11. Glasser, Ronald J. 1998. The Doctor is Not In. *Harper's Magazine* **296** (1774): 35.
12. Lee, Paul. 1995. A Plant is not a Factory. In *Proceedings of the 1st Wholistic Scientific Aromatherapy Conference,* Schnaubelt, K. (ed), 45-62. Pacific Institute of Aromatherapy, San Rafael.
13. Illich, Ivan. 1976. *Medical Nemesis: The Expropriation of Health.* Pantheon Books, New York.
14. Evans, Nancy. 1998. Medical journal loses credibility. Editorial in San Francisco Examiner, January 26.

Chapter Two

1. Rovesti, Paolo. 1995. *Auf der Suche nach den verlorenen Düften.* Irisiana, München.
2. *ibid.,* 19-21.
3. Grisanti, E. P. 1993. The Challenges of a United Europe for the Flavor and Fragrance Industry. *Perfumer & Flavorist* **18** (1): 1-7.
4. Saumäβiger Kohldampf. 1994. *Der Spiegel* **48**: 214-218. Hamburg.
5. Tyrrel, Michael. 1995. Advances in Natural Flavors and Materials. *Perfumer & Flavorist* **20** (1): 13-21.
6. See for instance the recent success of 'White Truffle Oil', which comes at a substantial price for a small quantity, yet the product is synthetic.
7. Marquez, Gabriel Garcia. 1988. *Love in the Time of Cholera.* Alfred A. Knopf, New York.
8. Süβkind, Patrick. 1985. *Das Parfüm.* Diogenes, ZÅrich.
   —Robbins, Tom. 1984. *Jitterbug Perfume.* Bantam Books, New York.
9. For instance in the now famous company name "Industrial Light and Magic."
10. Albone, Eric S. and Natynczuk. Stephan E. 1992. Mammals and Semiochemicals. In *Fragrance. The Psychology and Biology of Perfume,* van Toler, S., and Dodd, G.H. (eds), 63-69. Elsevier Applied Science. London.

11. Labows, J.N. and Preti, G. 1992. Human Semiochemicals. In *Fragrance: The Psychology and Biology of Perfumery,* van Toller, S. and Dodd, G. H. (eds), 69-88. Elsevier Science Publishers Ltd. Essex.
   —Ohloff, Günther. 1992. *Irdische Düfte Himmlische Lust: Eine Kulturgeschichte der Duftstoffe.* 14 -16. Birkhäuser Verlag, Basel.
12. Baydar, A. E., Petrzilka, M., Schott, M.P. 1992. Perception of Characteristic Axillary Odor. In *Proceedings of the 12th International Congress of Flavors, Fragrances and Essential Oils,* Woidich, H. and Buchbauer, G. (eds), 427-441. Vienna: Austrian Assoc. Flav. Fragr. Industry.
13. Schleidt, M. 1992. The Semiotic Relevance of Human Olfaction: A Biological Approach. In *Perfumery: The Psychology and Biology of Fragrance,* van Toller, S. and Dodd, G. H. (eds), 37. Elsevier Science Publishers Ltd. Essex.

Chapter Three

1. Frohne, D. and Jensen, U. 1992. *Systematik des Pflanzenreichs.* Gustav Fischer, Stuttgart.
2. Tétényi, P. 1975. Polychemismus bei ätherischölhaltigen Pflanzenarten. *Planta Medica* **28**: 230-243.
3. Tudge, Colin. 1996. *The Time Before History.* Simon and Schuster, NY.
4. Pert, Candace B. 1997. *Molecules of Emotion.* Scribner, New York.
5. Francke, W. 1991. Semiochemicals: Mevalogenins in Systems of Chemical Communication. In *Perfumes, Art Science Technology,* Müller, P.M. and Lamparsky, D. (eds), 61-100. Elsevier, London.
6. Lembke, A. und Deininger, R. 1987. Wirkung von Terpenen auf mikroskopische Pilze, Bakterien und Viren. In *Phytotherapie: Grundlagen, Klinik, Praxis,* Reuter, H.D. Deininger, and Schulz, V. (eds), 90-104. Hippokrates, Stuttgart.

Chapter Four

1. Buchbauer, G. 1995. Methods in Aromatherapy Research. In *Proceedings of the 13th International Congress of Flavors, Fragrances and Essential Oils, Istanbul, Turkey,* Baser, K.H.C. (ed), **3**, 80-89. Anadolu University Press, Eskisehir, Turkey.
2. Hendrickson, J. B., Cram, D. J., and Hammond, G. S. 1970. *Organic Chemistry,* 1—3, McGraw-Hill Book Company, New York.
3. Buchbauer, G. and Jirovetz, L. 1994. Aromatherapy—Use of Fragrances and Essential Oils as Medicaments. *Flavour & Fragrance, J.* **9**: 217-222.

4. Kawasaki, M. 1990. The Psychophysiological Effects of Odors, Aromachology. *Koryo* **168**: 43; Translated by Takasago Intern. Corp. 1-14.
5. Torii, S., Fukuda, H., Kanemoto, H., Miyauchi, R., Hamauzu, Y., and Kawasaki, M. 1988. Contingent Negative Variation (CNV) and the Psychological Effects of Odour. In *Perfumery: The Psychology and Biology of Fragrance,* van Toller, S. and Dodd, G.H. (eds), 107-120. Chapman & Hall, London.
6. Kubota, M., Ikemoto, T., Komaki, R. and Inui, M. 1992. Psychology of Perfume. In *Proceedings of the 12th International Congress of Flavors, Fragrances and Essential Oils,* Woidich, H. and Buchbauer, G. (eds), 456-461.Vienna: Austrian Assoc. Flav. Fragr. Industry.
7. Konishi H. et al. 1989. Japanese Cosmet. Sci. Soc. **3**, 140 cited according to ref. 4.
8. Jellinek, J.S. 1994. Aroma-Chology: A Status Review. *Perfumer & Flavorist* **19** (5): 25.
9. Guthrie, Helen. 1997. Close Encounters of the Essential Kind; A Case for Khella. *Aromatherapy Quarterly* **54**: 37.
10. Aflatoxin is a metabolic product of the fungus Aspergillus flavus, which is toxic to the liver and carcinogenic. See Wagner, Hildebert. 1993. *Pharmazeutische Biologie, Drogen und ihre Inhaltsstoffe, 5th Ed.,* 263. Gustav Fischer, Stuttgart.
11. Minski, Robyn. 1997. Letter to the Editor. *Simply Essential* **25**: 5.
12. Hephrun, Bernie. 1997. Aromatherapy—Quo Vadis? Presented at VEROMA Aromatherapy Conference. Zug, Switzerland, Oct. 4.
    —Watt, Martin. 1997. Letter to the Editor. *The Aromatic Thymes.* **5** (3): 6.
13. Lee, Paul. 1995. A Plant is not a Factory. In *First Wholistic Scientific Aromatherapy Conference Proceedings,* K. Schnaubelt (ed), 45-61. Pacific Institute of Aromatherapy, San Rafael.

Chapter Five

1. Roszak, Theodore. 1992. *The Voice of the Earth.* Simon & Schuster, New York.
    —Roszak, Theodore. 1986. *The Cult of Information.* Pantheon Books, New York.
    —Roszak, Theodore. 1995. *The Memoirs of Elizabeth Frankenstein.* Bantam Books, New York.

2. Spretnak, Charlene. 1997. *Resurgence of the Real.* Addison-Wesley Publishing Company, New York.
3. Laurence, Leslie and Weinhouse, Beth. 1994. *Outrageous Practices.* Fawcett Columbine, New York.
4. *ibid.,* 121.
5. *ibid.,.* 126.
6. *ibid.,* 171.
7. *ibid.,* 223.
8. Max Weber. 1992. *The The Protestant Ethic and the Spirit of Capitalism.* Routledge, London and New York.
9. Schmidt, Michael; Smith, Lendon; Sehnert, Keith. 1993. *Beyond Antibiotics.* North Atlantic Books, Berkeley.
10. *ibid.,* 25.
11. Weil, Andrew. 1995. *Spontaneous Healing.* Alfred A. Knopf, New York.
12. Glasser, Ronald J. 1998. The Doctor is Not In. *Harper's Magazine* **296** (1774): 35.
    —Reich, Charles A. 1995. *Opposing the System.* Crown Publishers. New York.
13. Lowen, Rebecca S. 1997. *Creating the Cold War University: The Transformation of Stanford.* University of California Press.
14. See for instance Abstracts of the 2nd World Congress on Medicinal and Aromatic Plants for Human Welfare (WOPMAC II), Nov. 10-15 Mendoza, Argentina.
15. For instance Williams, Lyall R. et al. 1993. Antimicrobial Activity of Oil of Melaleuca (Tea Tree Oil). *Cosmetics, Aerosols & Toiletries* **4**: 4
16. A particularly obvious example for statements made without having any clue of the existing literature is Gates, R. Patrick. 1995. Aromatherapy: The Nose Knows, But Can the Nose Cure? *Alternative Medicine Journal* May/June **23**: 5-6. Prime National Publishing Corp. Weston, MA.
    —Another example of selecting just a few factoids is Lis-Balchin, Maria. 1995. *Aroma Science—The Chemistry and Bioactivity of Essential Oils.* Amberwood Publishing, East Horsley, Surrey, UK.
17. Moore, Thomas J. 1995. *Deadly Medicine.* Simon & Schuster, New York.
18. Illich, Ivan. 1976. *Medical Nemesis: The Expropriation of Health.* Pantheon Books, New York.
19. see ref. 12
20. Reich, Charles A. 1995. *Opposing the System.* Crown Publishers, New York.

21. Kaku, Michio. 1997. *Visions*. 192. Doubleday, New York.
22. Shiva, Vandana. 1988. Reductionist Science as Epistemological Violence. In *Science, Hegemony and Violence: A Requiem for Modernity*. Oxford University Press, New Dehli.
23. Nandy, Ashis. 1988. Science as the Reason of State. In *Science, Hegemony and Violence: A Requiem for Modernity*. Oxford University Press, New Dehli.
24. Appfel-Marglin, Frederique. 1993. Development or Decolonialization in the Andes. *Daybreak* **4** (3): 6-10.

Chapter Six

1. Tesseire, Paul Jose. 1994. *Chemistry of Fragrant Substances*. VCH Publishers, New York.
2. Hendrickson, J. B., Cram, D. J., and Hammond, G. S. 1970. *Organic Chemistry*. 1 - 3. McGraw-Hill Book Company, New York.
3. Gildemeister, E. and Hoffmann, Fr. 1956. *Die atherischen Öle*. Wilhelm Treibs (ed), Akademie Verlag, Berlin.
   —Guenther, Ernest. 1948. *The Essential Oils*. D. Van Nostrand Company, Inc. New York.
4. Adams, Robert, P. 1995. *Identification of Essential Oil Components by Gas Chromatography/Mass Spectroscopy*. Allured Publishing, Carol Stream, Il.
5. Kubeczka, K. H. (ed). 1979. In *Vorkommen und Analytik atherischer Öle, Ergebnisse Internationaler Arbeitstagungen in Würzburg, Freiburg und Münster*. Georg Thieme Verlag, Stuttgart, Germany.
6. *ibid.:* R. Hegnauer. Verbreitung ätherischer Öle im Pflanzenreich.
   —Kubeczka, Karl-Heinz. Possibilities of Quality Determination of Medicinally Used Essential Oils.
   —Heinrich, G. Zur Cytologie und Physiologie ätherischer Öle erzeugender pflanzlicher Drüsenzellen.
   —Rücker, G. Systematische Identifizierung und Strukturaufklärung von Sesquiterpenen.
7. Schilcher, H. 1982. Zur Analytik der Inhaltstoffe der Matricaria chamomilla L. In *Äétherischer Öle: Analytik, Physiologie, Zusammensetzung, Ergebnisse Internationaler Arbeitstagungen in Würzburg und Groningen,* Kubeczka, K.-H. (ed), 104–115. Georg Thieme Verlag, Stuttgart, Germany.
   —Baerheim-Svendsen, A. and Scheffer, J.J.C. (eds). 1985. *Essential Oils and Aromatic Plants, Proceedings of the 15th International Symposium on*

Essential Oils. Martinus Nijhoff, and Dr. W. Junk Publishers, The Netherlands.

8. Brunke, E. J. (ed). 1986. *Progress in Essential Oil Research, Proceedings of the International Symposium on Essential Oils, Holzminden/ Neuhaus*. Walter de Gruyter. Berlin. Germany.
9. *ibid.,* 99—110: Boelens, Mans H., and Jimenez Sindreu, Rafael. The chemical composition of Laurel leaf oil, obtained by steam distillation and hydrodiffusion.
10. *ibid.,* 177-196: Weyerstahl, P. et al. Isolation and synthesis of compounds from the essential oil of Helichrysum italicum.
11. *ibid.,* 429-448: Knobloch, K. et al. Action of terpenoids on energy metabolism.
12. Keller, W., Kober. 1955. W. *Arzneim. Forsch.* **5**, 224.
—Keller, W., Kober. 1955. W. *Arzneim. Forsch.* **6**, 768.
13. Wagner, H. and Sprinkmeyer, L. 1973. Über die pharmakologische Wirkung von Melissengeist. *Deutsche Apotheker Zeitung* **113**: 1159-1166.
14. Pellecuer, J., Allegrini, J. 1975. Place de l'essence de satureia montana L. dans l'arsenal therapeutique. *Plantes medicinales et phytothérapie* **IX** (2): 99-106.
15. Belaiche, Paul. 1979. *Traite de phytotherapie et d'aromatherapie.* Maloine S.A. Editeur, Paris.
16. Deininger, Rolf. 1975. Zentrale Wirkung der Terpene. *Erfahrungsheilkunde* **24** (10): 261-264.
17. Lembke, A. and Deininger. R. 1987. Wirkung von Terpenen auf mikroskopische Pilze, Bakterien und Viren. In *Phytotherapie: Grundlagen, Klinik, Praxis,* Reuter, H.D. Deininger, and Schulz, V. (eds), 90-104. Hippokrates, Stuttgart.
18. see ref. 13.
19. Hammer, O. 1974. Wirkungsnachweis zur therapeutischen Anwendung von Terpenen. *Folia phytotherapeutica* **6**: 4.
20. Büchner. K., Hellings, H., Huber, M., Peukert, E., Späth, L., Deininger, R. 1974. *Medizinische Klinik* **69**: 1032-1036. Urban & Schwarzenberg.
21. Lingen, K.H. 1974. Über die therapeutische Wirksamkeit von Melissengeist bei psychovegetativen Syndromen. *die heilkunst* **87** (2): 1-3.
22. Deininger, Rolf. 1995. The Spectrum of Activity of Plant Drugs Containing Essential Oils (Especially their Antibacterial, Antifungal and Antiviral Activity). In *Proceedings of the First Wholistic Scientific Aromatherapy Conference,* Schnaubelt, Kurt (ed), 15-43. Pacific Institute of Aromatherapy, San Rafael, CA.

23. *ibid.*, 23.
24. Schumacher, E. F. 1975. *Small is Beautiful—Economics as if People Mattered.* Harper Perennial, New York.
25. Johard, U., Eklund, A., Hed, J., Lundahl, J. 1993. Terpenes enhance metabolic activity and alter expression of adhesion molecules (Mac-1 and L-selectin) on human granulocytes. *Inflammation* **17** (4): 499-509.
26. Jirtle, Randy L., Haag, Jill D., Ariazi, Eric A., Gould, Michael N. 1993. Increased mannose 6-phosphate/insulin-like growth factor II receptor and transforming growth factor beta 1 levels during monoterpene-induced regression of mammary tumors. *Cancer Res.* **53** (17): 3849-52.
   —Gould, M.N. 1995. Prevention of mammary cancer by monoterpenes. Journal of Cellular Biochemistry 22: 139-44.
27. Erreira, F., Santos, M.S., Faro, C., Pires, E., Carvalho, A.P., Cunha, A.P., Macedo, T. 1996. Effects of Valeriana officinalis on [3H] GABA. Release in synaptosomes: further evidence for the involvement of free GABA in the Valerian-induced release. *Rev. Port. Farm.* **46** (2): 74-77.
   —Cavadas, C., Araujo, I., Cotrim, M.D., Amaral, T., Cunha, A.P. 1995. In vitro study on the interaction of Valeriana officinalis L. extracts and their amino acids on GABA receptor in rat brain. *Arzneim—Forsch.* **45** (7): 753-5.
28. Elisabetsky, E. 1997. Anticonvulsant Properties of Linalool and gamma-decanolactone in Mice. WOCMAP II - Abstracts, Mendoza, Argentina.
29. Dolara, Piero; Moneti, Gloriano; Pieraccini, Giuseppe; Romanelli, Novella. 1996. Characterization of the action on central opioid receptors of furaneudesma-1,3-diene, a sesquiterpene extracted from myrrh. *Phytother. Re.* **10**, Suppl. 1: 81-83.
30. Rao, Renee C. 1994. et al. Khusimol, a non-peptide ligand for vasopressin V1a receptors. *J. Nat. Prod.* **57** (10): 1329-35.
31. Illes, George P. et al. 1976. Synthesis of a bioactive compounds. A structure-activity study of aryl terpenes as juvenile hormone mimics. *J. Agric. Food Chem.* **24** (4): 699-708.
32. Cornwell, P.A., Barry, B.W. 1994. Sesquiterpene components of volatile oils as skin penetration enhancers for hydrophilic permeant 5-florouracil. *J. Pharm. Pharmacol.* **46** (4): 261-9.

Chapter Seven

1. Schnaubelt, Kurt. 1995. Essential Oils: Viable Wholistic Pharmaceuticals for the Future. In *Proceedings of the 13th International Congress of Fla-*

vors, Fragrances and Essential Oils, Istanbul, Turkey, Baser, K.H.C. (ed), **3**, 269-281. Anadolu University Press, Eskisehir, Turkey.

—You, Brenda. 1994. *Is aromatherapy a cure-all right under our noses?* Chicago Tribune March 29.

2. Dürbeck, K. and Wildner, A. 1991. Handelsförderung von Extrakten aus Arznei und Gewürzpflanzen sowie Phytopharmaka. Entwicklung und ländlicher Raum **4**: 18-19.

   —Dürbeck, K., Wildner, A. 1992. H. Trade Promotion of Medicinal and Aromatic Plant Products—a PROTRADE offer to developing countries' producers. In *Proceedings of the First World Congress On Medicinal And Aromatic Plants For Human Welfare (WOPMAC),* Franz, Ch., Seitz, R., Verlet, N. (eds), 55. Maastricht, Netherlands.

3. see Capitalistic Bureaucracies. In Reich, Charles A. 1995. *Opposing the System.* Crown Publishers, New York.

   —Hall, Carl T. 1998. *Magic Elixir for Drug Sales.* San Francisco Chronicle, March 12, E1. San Francisco, CA.

   —Tucker, Cynthia. 1995. The Unprofitability of Healthcare. Editorial San Francisco Chronicle.

4. Moore, Thomas J. 1955. *Deadly Medicine.* Simon & Schuster, New York.
5. Düsberg, Peter. 1994. *Inventing the Aids Virus.* Regnery Publishing, New York.

   —The Assault on David Baltimore. May 1996. *The New Yorker.*

6. Kaku, Michio. 1997. *Visions.* Doubleday, New York.
7. Special Report Winter 1996. 1996. *Taipan.* Baltimore, MD.
8. Neviodow, Leo A. 1996. *Der Sechste Kondratieff.* Rhein-Sieg Verlag, Sankt Augustin, Germany
9. *ibid.,* 120.

Chapter Eight

1. Schmidt, Michael; Smith, Lendon; Sehnert, Keith. 1993. *Beyond Antibiotics.* North Atlantic Books, Berkeley.
2. Langbein, Kurt, Martin Hans-Peter et al. 1981. *Gesunde Geschäfte.* Kiepenheuer und Witsch, Köln.

Chapter Nine

1. Deininger, Rolf. 1995. The Magic World of Essential Oils and Scents: Their Effect on the Psyche. In *Proceedings of the 1st Wholistic Scientific*

Aromatherapy Conference, Schnaubelt, K. (ed), 90-113. Pacific Institute of Aromatherapy, San Rafael.

2. Deininger, Rolf. 1995. The Spectrum of Activity of Plant Drugs Containing Essential Oils (Especially their Antibacterial, Antifungal and Antiviral Activity). In *Proceedings of the 1st Wholistic Scientific Aromatherapy Conference,* Schnaubelt, K. (ed), 15-43. Pacific Institute of Aromatherapy, San Rafael.
3. Headline Story in San Francisco Chronicle from the New York Times. 1998, April 15: Warning on Deadly Drug Side Effects: Study Says Medications Kill Over 100,000 a Year. San Francisco.
4. Garret, Laurie. 1994. *The Coming Plague: New Emerging Diseases in a World out of Balance.* Farrar, Straus and Giroux, New York.
5. Evans, Nancy. 1998. Medical journal loses credibility. Editorial in San Francisco Examiner, January 26.
6. Guitton, Jean, Bogdanov Grischka and Igor. 1993. *Gott und die Wissenschaft: Auf dem Weg zum Metarealismus.* München.
7. Zimmer, E. Dieter. 1981. *Die Vernunft der Gefühle. Ursprung und Sinn der menschlichen Emotion.* München.
   —Podak, Klaus. 1998. Leben heiβt Zeichen Geben. Süddeutschen Zeitung, **61**. München, Germany.
8. Wall, Steve. 1994. *Shadowcatchers.* Harper Collins Publishers, New York.
9. *ibid.*
10. *ibid.*
11. Schumacher, E. F. 1975. *Small is Beautiful: Economics as if People Mattered.* Harper Perennial, New York.

Chapter Ten

1. International Organization for Stadardization, Geneva.
2. Denny, E.F.K. 1987. *Field Distillation for Herbaceous Oils.* Tasmania.
   —Wijesekera, R.O.B., Ratnatung, C.M., and Dürbeck K. 1997. *The Distillation of Essential Oils.* Protrade, Deutsche Gesellschaft für Technische Zusammenarbeit. Eschborn, Germany.
3. Rovesti, Paolo. 1995. *Auf der Suche nach den verlorenen Düften.* Irisiana, München.
4. Brunschwig. approx. 1500. Liber de Arte Distillandi. Strasbourg.
   —Theophrastus. 1556. De Odoribus. Paris.
5. Kubeczka, Karl-Heinz. 1979. Possibilities of Quality Determination of Medicinally Used Essential Oils. In *Vorkommen und Analytik Ätherischer*

Öle, Ergebnisse Internationaler Arbeitstagungen in Würzburg, Freiburg und Münster. Georg Thieme Verlag, Stuttgart.

Chapter Eleven

1. Joulain, D. 1994. Methods for analyzing essential oils: Modern analysis methodologies, uses and abuses. *Perfumer & Flavorist* **19** (2): 5-17.
2. Wagner, Hildebert. 1993. *Pharmazeutische Biologie, Drogen und ihre Inhaltsstoffe, 5th Ed.* Gustav Fischer, Stuttgart.
   —Schnaubelt, Kurt. 1985. *The Aromatherapy Course.* Pacific Institute of Aromatherapy, San Rafael.
3. König, W.A., Rieck, A., Fricke, C., Melching, S., Saritas, Y. and Hardt, I.H. 1995. Enantiomeric Composition of Sesquiterpenes in Essential Oils. In *Proceedings of the 13th International Congress of Flavors, Fragrances and Essential Oils, Istanbul, Turkey,* Baser, K.H.C. (ed), **2**, 169. Anadolu University Press, Eskisehir, Turkey.
   —Mosandl, Armin. 1993. Neue methoden zur herkunftsspezifischen Analyse ätherischer Öle. In Ätherische Öle, Anspruch und Wirklichkeit, Carle, Reinhold (ed) 103-134. Wissenschaftliche Verlagsgesellschaft mbH, Stuttgart.
4. Brunke, E. J. and Schmaus, G. 1995. Trace Constituents of Sensory Importance—Recent Results. In *Proceedings of the 13th International Congress of Flavors, Fragrances and Essential Oils, Istanbul, Turkey,* Baser, K.H.C. (ed), **3**, 186. Anadolu University Press, Eskisehir, Turkey.
5. Boelens, M.H. 1995. Chemical & Sensory Evaluation of Trace Compounds in Naturals. In *Proceedings of the 13th International Congress of Flavors, Fragrances and Essential Oils, Istanbul, Turkey,* Baser, K.H.C. (ed), 3, 177. Anadolu University Press, Eskisehir, Turkey.
6. Ford, Richard A. 1991. The Toxicology and Safety of Fragrances. In *Perfumes, Art Science Technology,* Müller, P.M. and Lamparsky, D. (eds), 441-463. Elsevier, London.
7. Mrasek, Volker. 1998. Duftstoffe die unter die Haut gehen. *Süddeutsche Zeitung,* January 22, München, Germany.

Chapter Twelve

1. Schnaubelt, Kurt. 1998. *Advanced Aromatherapy.* Healing Arts Press, Rochester VT.
   —Schnaubelt, Kurt. 1985. *The Aromatherapy Course.* Pacific Institute of Aromatherapy, San Rafael.

2. Mazza, Giacomo. 1987. Identification of new compounds in citrus oils by GC/MS. *Essenze Deriv. Agrum.* **57** (1): 19-33.

Chapter Thirteen

1. Haas, Monika and Schnaubelt, Kurt. 1992. Breathing Space. *The International Journal of Aromatherapy* **4** (4): 13-15.

Epilogue

1. Ohloff, Günther. 1992. *Irdische DüÅfte Himmlische Lust: Eine Kulturgeschichte der Duftstoffe* 21. Birkhäuser Verlag, Basel.
   —Deininger, Rolf. 1993. Duft und Psyche: Der Einfluβ des Duftes auf die Psyche des Menschen. *Zeitschrift fur Phytotherapie* **14:** 193-205. Stuttgart, Germany.

Index

B

C

F

G

N

R

Kurt Schnaubelt earned his Ph.D. in Germany from Technical University of Munich. A leader in aromatherapy in the United States since 1983, he is the author of *Advanced Aromatherapy*, a textbook on scientifically based aromatherapy originally published in Cologne in 1995. He is scientific director of the Pacific Institute of Aromatherapy, an educational and research organization which sponsors international conventions on aromatherapy, and is founder and CEO of Original Swiss Aromatics in San Rafael, California.